Understanding Breast Cancer Risk

Patricia T. Kelly

Temple University Press
Philadelphia

Temple University Press, Philadelphia 19122

Published 1991
Printed in the United States of America

The paper used in this publication meets the minimum requirements of American National Standard for Information Sciences—Permanence of Paper for Printed Library Materials, ANSI Z39.48-1984 ∞

Library of Congress Cataloging-in-Publication Data
Kelly, Patricia T., 1942–
Understanding breast cancer risk / Patricia T. Kelly.
p. cm.—(Health, society, and policy)
Includes bibliographical references and index.
ISBN 0-87722-812-4 (cloth : alk. paper)—
ISBN 0-87722-813-2 (pbk. : alk. paper)
1. Breast—Cancer—Risk factors. I. Title. II. Series.
[DNLM: 1. Breast Neoplasms. 2. Risk Factors. WP 870 K29u]
RC280.B8K45 1991
616.99'449071—dc20
DNLM/DLC
for Library of Congress 90-11237

To Jena and Sean

Contents

List of Figures

List of Tables

Acknowledgments

Information presented in *Understanding Breast Cancer Risk* was gathered over a period of more than ten years while I worked with concerned individuals and families. They taught me the range of significant topics and how to present each in a more meaningful fashion. Without the courage and honest communication of these forthright individuals, the field of Breast Cancer Risk Analysis could not have come into being.

As the scope, importance, and role of Breast Cancer Risk Analysis was first becoming clear to me, I was given great encouragement and support by Doctors Thomas K. Hunt, Mary-Claire King, Nicholas L. Petrakis, Ernest H. Rosenbaum, Sheryl Ruzek, and Irving K. Zola.

I am grateful for comments and suggestions on this manuscript made by my colleagues, Doctors David E. Anderson, John C. Arpels, Philip B. Kivitz, Michael D. Lagios, Frederick R. Margolin, Robert C. Nachtigall, Mark C. Rounsaville, Rodger M. Shepherd, Gilbert A. Webb, and by nurse Cathy Coleman, who also provided valuable assistance in the compilation of Appendix B. Librarians Lydia Jensen and Peggy Tahir greatly aided my search for relevant studies. My editors, Sheryl Ruzek and Janet M. Francendese, provided a thoughtful analysis of the manuscript as a whole as well as a valuable critique of individual chapters.

Understanding Breast Cancer Risk

Introduction: The Book, Its Audience and Purpose

> It's a tug between the hysterical part of you that doesn't want to know, and the rational part that wants to do more than worry.

As a medical geneticist who provides breast cancer risk assessment and counseling, I am accustomed to hearing women express their anxiety about breast cancer. In the course of risk analysis, I find that for most, the risk of breast cancer is far lower than they had expected. Many patients tell me they are confused about risk information available in the public media and are unsure about how to ask their questions; they also worry that they might not be in the appropriate specialist's office to raise their particular concerns. These women—and many others—need greater access to and understanding of the new risk information now available, as well as help in applying it to their own lives and health care practices. This book addresses the questions and concerns patients frequently raise as they seek information regarding their individual risks and appropriate breast health care and treatment.

Breast Cancer Risk Analysis makes use of information from the fields of genetics, medicine, epidemiology, sociology, and counseling. Its aim is to provide clear, relevant information to concerned women and to help them make decisions about treatment options and breast health care based on this information. As a specialist in the evaluation of studies on breast cancer risk and treatment, I analyze an individual's risk of this disease and discuss my findings with her and her health care providers. In over ten years of clinical practice, in previous experience in research genetics at the University of California, San Francisco, and in teaching graduate students at the University of California, Berkeley, I developed a great deal of valuable information for those interested in understanding and communicating information about breast cancer risk.

The Audience

This book is written for health professionals who provide care to women with a breast concern—some focusing on nursing and medicine, others specializing in the educational, social, and psychological aspects of patient care. It is designed to help health professionals more clearly understand: the extent of scientific information currently available on a wide range of factors often associated with breast cancer risk; the evaluation of studies and the relevance of study results and statistics to patients; and effective means of communicating risk information to patients. (For convenience, those who seek a health professional's care or advice are called patients in this book.)

In my practice, I am often asked about the effects of age, benign breast disease, reproductive history, family history, diet, stress, personality, hormones, and other factors on a woman's risk of breast cancer. Of course, women want more than just a number; they want also to understand their risk so they can devise a health program that will give them peace of mind while reducing their chances of dying or losing a breast. This book addresses such concerns, but cannot include all the background information or summarize all the research on breast cancer risk—nor can it provide the expertise necessary to develop a formal risk analysis or counseling approach to breast cancer risk.

Writing for a diverse audience has led to certain compromises in content and approach, sometimes resulting in simplistic generalizations. I hope that specialists in each field will realize the importance of presenting elementary concepts of their area to others, and will appreciate that these concepts are intended for health professionals with differing specialties. This book has been written for health professionals, yet patients and their families may also wish to use the information presented here as a basis for discussing their individual circumstances with health professionals.

Health professionals who see patients with a breast concern or breast cancer need to be able to interpret study results and clearly convey this information to patients. For this reason, I have included the specific results of many studies as well as guides for interpreting these results. Means of communicating information about risk are also given, since the aim is to help patients understand and make use of it.

Many patients are quite naturally bewildered by changes in medical and scientific findings on breast cancer risk. One plaintively asked: "Why are we told one year that birth control pills or fibrocystic disease increase risk, and the next year that they don't? How can I ever make sense of it all?" As I will show, careful analysis of earlier studies would have led to caution in interpreting the results—a caution I advise in analyzing studies of today. Each scientific study must be analyzed in terms of its strengths and weaknesses and in the context of results obtained from similar studies.

In general, I recognize a particular risk factor as clinically important only when a group of studies clearly suggests that this factor is associated with increased risk. Other health professionals may have a lower threshold of acceptance. In this book, I present sufficient information about a number of studies so readers can judge the reliability of results for themselves.

Need for This Book

The need for a book on breast cancer risk has increased in recent years as women have become more interested in health and disease prevention and are participating more fully in making decisions about their own medical care. In recent years also, new and often conflicting information has been widely reported in the mass media, confusing many women about the relevance of various risk factors to their own lives. Women confronted with conflicting medical opinions, confusing information, and the emotional stress that often accompanies uncertainty about cancer risk, quite naturally feel an increased need for clear and precise information to enable them to make decisions about their breast health care and treatment.

Some health professionals express concern that information, particularly information given at a stressful time, will increase patient confusion. Instead, I find confusion and anxiety often result when a patient has too little information, or insufficient information about a particular topic. Patients frequently lack the expertise to identify what information is needed to make sense of a given situation, and so rely on health professionals to discover and supply missing pieces. In my experience, patients rarely use information about breast cancer risk to make inappropriate medical decisions. Instead, a search for information and clarification, even if prolonged, usually signifies that an individual has not yet been able to make sense of what she has heard. In one study, for example, cancer patients were found to want physicians to make medical decisions and to provide more information (Sutherland et al. 1989).

Overview

Chapter 1 is a compendium of women's beliefs about breast cancer etiology, risk, and treatment and identifies some of the social and psychological barriers that can impede a patient's understanding of information. A sampling of the special reactions and considerations of women whose mothers had breast cancer are presented here also.

A guide to interpreting studies and risk information is presented in Chapter 2. This chapter is particularly important since it establishes a standard language and methodology used in discussing study results presented throughout the book. I note misconceptions that can arise when patients are given relative risk information instead of numerical risks, or when they fail to appreciate the difference between risks that are increased and those that are increased but not large. This chapter presents other statistical and methodological issues clearly and simply.

Chapter 3 is devoted to a discussion of benign breast disease (fibrocystic disease) and the in situ breast cancers. It describes the risk of breast cancer associated with each of these different cell types and the treatment options available. Chapter 4 summarizes studies on risk factors of frequent concern to patients, including diet, stress, and reproductive history. Chapter 5 considers the effects of hormones taken for birth control or at menopause on a woman's breast cancer risk. Studies pertaining to DES exposure and breast cancer risk are also reviewed.

Chapter 6 discusses risk to women who have a family history of breast cancer. Some fundamentals of genetics, a brief description of oncogenes and the new Restriction Fragment Length Polymorphism (RFLP) tests are included in a discussion of advances in this rapidly changing field.

Chapter 7 summarizes the results of recent studies on breast cancer detection and includes guidelines my patients have found useful in dealing with a breast concern. This chapter is designed to help health professionals to educate and counsel patients who are confused or uneasy about their future breast health care or treatment.

1

The Patient's Perspective

An individual's beliefs about the origin, treatment, and prognosis of breast cancer may prevent her from seeking or understanding information about risk, treatment options, or the improved prognoses expected with early disease detection. Therefore, health professionals will find it most valuable to learn about patients' breast cancer beliefs—that is, how they define this disease. Such information can rarely be obtained quickly or in a straightforward manner, since individuals often are unaware of their beliefs in this regard.

For example, a woman often views a friend's or a relative's experience with breast cancer as the usual or even the only disease course. If someone she knew died of breast cancer, she may equate the disease with death. One woman whose mother died of breast cancer assumed that the disease would be fatal to her also, saying:

> I'm child-oriented, very much like my mother. And when I think of not living to see my children a little bit older . . . [cries]. I feel that I'm the only one who can raise them the right way. Leaving them is what frightens me.

Women whose friend or relative had treatments no longer in use frequently equate these outmoded methods with modern treatments. Individuals may realize intellectually that improved treatments are now available, but continue to remember and to dread the disease as experienced by their friend or relative.

A great deal can be learned about a person's beliefs by listening carefully to descriptions of her own, her relatives', and her friends' experiences with medical problems, especially those involving the breast. If a patient feels comfortable describing these experiences during the first visit, I find it most worthwhile to listen. To avoid patients rambling, I ask questions to help move the story along or to deepen my understanding of their view of a given situation. If the events happened some time ago, I find it useful to elicit a description of how they felt then and how they feel now. Many, after hearing their own responses, say they hadn't realized how their feelings had changed. For example, anger and fear are often reduced over time, particularly if the individual was a child when the friend or relative was affected. In some cases, these feelings have increased as individuals learned more about what might have been done to help a loved one. It is the process of speaking about the events that often brings greater clarity and understanding.

Beliefs About Causes of Cancer

There are almost as many beliefs about the causes of breast cancer as there are people. It is important to learn how and when your patient believes breast cancer occurs so you can correct misinformation and better help her to understand the most recent scientific thinking. The following are examples of the range of beliefs about cause. There are many others, of course.

Some feel cancer results from a spontaneous change in a cell that causes it to "explode," "get out of line," or "go its own way." Friction, rubbing, and trauma are also thought to cause breast cancer. In fact, some women are reluctant to examine their own breasts for fear of causing disease or bringing about a spread. Some worry about the time they hit their breast on a steering wheel, an object fell from a closet, or a baby kicked them on the breast. Some fear that breast cancer is contagious. For example, one woman said, "If you're not too strong, you can catch cancer from someone else." Another said, "I drank out of my stepfather's cup when he was dying of lung cancer, so perhaps my cancer risk is increased."

Many believe an individual's psychological state either causes breast cancer or significantly increases susceptibility to the disease. (For a review of scientific studies in this area, see Chapter 4.) Some are afraid that even thinking about cancer might act as a cause. As one of my patients said:

> Fear of cancer can cause cancer. We mentally make ourselves susceptible and that makes us physically susceptible. Thinking creates one's destiny.

Some believe individuals who develop cancer have an inability to love:

> They say that if you get breast cancer, you are the kind of person who is unable to receive love, so breast cancer puts you in a place where you have to receive it. You become really helpless, and you have to depend on others and receive from them.

To some, cancer is associated with a lowered resistance due to illness, the death of a loved one, or a feeling of depression. Women remember when they or a relative were not feeling well, and ascribe the onset of breast cancer to that time. In such cases, it is important to help patients understand that it generally takes years for breast cancer to grow, so depression six months before a diagnosis is unlikely to have resulted in cancer.

It is not unusual for patients to believe that a misdeed can cause breast cancer. Some feel guilty about injections they received to curtail lactation after childbirth, their poor diet, or even an abortion. Women dissatisfied with the size or shape of their breasts may also worry:

> When I found my lump, I had been planning breast augmentation. Right away I thought God was punishing me for not being satisfied with what I had.

I find it useful to spend the time to uncover women's beliefs about the causes of breast cancer since these beliefs may suggest issues that need to be stressed or pieces of information that need to be explained. The aim is not to dissuade patients from deeply cherished beliefs. Instead, it is to prevent erroneous beliefs from interfering with their comprehension of relevant information and the implementation of appropriate health practices.

Finding a Breast Lump

The depth of a woman's concerns about breast cancer can often be detected in the way she describes finding a lump or a change in the breast. Reactions vary greatly, of course, and are influenced by many personal and family experiences. Once a woman finds a breast change, she may wait before seeking a medical opinion. Some hope the questionable area will disappear:

> I knew I had a lump in my breast. But then I guess I hoped that I'd made a mistake and that the next time it would be gone.

Others say they keep forgetting about it, or postpone a visit to the doctor or nurse to avoid what might lie ahead:

> I was afraid I would have to make a big decision about whether to lose a breast or to die.

> If you don't report a lump, you can feel you still have options. You can kid yourself about it. You still have the

> option of thinking it's nothing. Once you go and find what it is, then you're there with the facts and you have to make a decision about it.

Often, women put family events before their own medical care. Many say they postponed a physician's appointment until the family moved, the children went off to summer camp, their husband's job project was well under way, and so forth. These are all ways to avoid facing the big changes that might occur in their own and their family's lives if they were found to have breast cancer. When viewed in this perspective, it is no wonder women hesitate.

Even women with great concerns about breast cancer tell of finding a breast change, promptly making an appointment to see a health professional, but failing to mention the lump or thickening while in the office. Some say they forgot to mention it. Others worry their physician or nurse will think they are hypochondriacs if they express the deep concern they feel when they think a change has occurred. In these cases, a woman may wait to see what the health professional finds:

> I thought if the lump was anything, the doctor would find it and mention it. He didn't say anything, so I thought there was nothing wrong. I told the new doctor I went to a few months later about it because it was still there. Plus, I felt more comfortable with him and felt he would take the time to examine me thoroughly.

Those whose relative died of breast cancer may feel especially threatened by the presence of a breast change:

> When I found my lump, I ran through the alternatives: dying, leaving my husband, biopsy, and so forth. I alternated between feeling I've had a good life and feeling it's unjust. I talked to my husband about leaving him if I had breast cancer, because I didn't want to put him through that. He said he would want to stay with me until the end. But then, he's never been through it.

As these examples illustrate, a woman's reactions to a breast lump may reveal a great deal about her concern level and her methods of coping. Therefore, it is well worth taking the time to learn how a previous experience may have affected her, and how she responded to it.

Coping with Fear and Concern

The way in which a woman copes with her concern about breast cancer may provide valuable information about how to help her achieve effective breast health care (see Chapter 7). Some cope by keeping busy:

> I keep my mind occupied with other things. Right now I've got a ninety-seven-hour-a-day job just trying to keep things under control in the business. Or I sew or do something else that I can get involved in.

Others attempt to think positively, hoping that this will protect them:

> I've set my mind that cancer is not for me. I don't intend to get it.

> I think wellness, not illness. I'm always looking forward to how well I'm going to be.

Some cope by finding a health professional who gives them hope:

> The main thing I've done has been to seek out someone who would say, 'In my best judgment, you're O.K.' And I've cast about a bit for that. That's the process that I've gone through until I've felt that I'd done my best to find the people I felt would give me the best chance, who did the most, and who had the most experiences that would

> be available to me. Once I had done that, then I felt more comfortable than I have ever been before.

Unfortunately, many do not realize what they should seek in a health professional and are not clear about what would reduce their anxiety or make them feel protected, and so they do not institute an adequate follow-up program for breast health care.

Some women experience anxiety about breast cancer on a regular basis. For example, one said:

> If it ever comes up I push it out of my head. But it's always underlying, it's always there. It's a very familiar thought. It pops up and you push it back down and it pops up.

Others associate even minor health problems with breast cancer:

> Whenever there's a problem with my health, I think about my breasts first. I don't have it on my mind all the time and it doesn't always keep me from sleeping, but it is always there in the background, waiting for me to worry about.

In my experience, those who find a breast health center in addition to excellent breast health professionals tend to cope better than those who do not.

Of course, not all of women's concerns about breasts have their origin in the fear of breast cancer. This important insight was clarified for me by a patient who is a psychiatrist. As she said:

> I've become increasingly aware that often my anxiety isn't particularly anxiety about my breasts. Often, when I'm getting worried about my breasts, it's a signal to me that something else is going on and that maybe something else isn't getting taken care of. If I take a look at my whole life situation, I can often discover that I am under some other kind of pressure. When I pay more attention to that pres-

sure, that will often help take care of my concern about breast cancer.

I find this displacement anxiety most frequently in women who have had a close friend or relative with breast or other cancer.

Risk Perceptions

It is important to determine a woman's assessment of her own breast cancer risk, since this often provides clear information about her level of concern. In some cases, individuals have a specific numerical risk in mind, in some cases not. Even when a patient uses a specific risk figure, I try to learn what this number means to her, and whether this is an emotional or intellectual assessment.

I am often asked by patients and health professionals about the value of risk assessment or of telling a woman her risk. After all, some say, a woman will either develop breast cancer or she won't. Obviously, risk analysis and giving patients information about risk factors does not affect risk of developing breast cancer. However, information about risk often influences the patient's choice of a breast health care program, the follow-up schedule physicians decide to institute, and the way in which women think about their lives. Risk information, in combination with the other information provided by Breast Cancer Risk Analysis, can do much to improve a woman's health care and quality of life.

Patients who initially say they are not interested in risk information often change their minds when they realize some of the ways in which all of us use probabilities to shape our daily lives. I remind them that most people use a seat belt to reduce risk of harm, not prevent it. In the same way, one can use probabilities to devise health programs that increase the chance of early detection should breast cancer occur. Additionally, most women gain an added sense of security by learning about various risk factors and basing their follow-up care on these findings.

Of course, women who have had unfortunate life experiences with breast cancer are more likely to feel emotionally threatened by this disease than those who have not had such experiences. To illustrate this increased sensitivity I sometimes use the example of a person who has been mugged in a safe neighborhood. All the neighbors say, "Oh, that couldn't possibly happen here again. It was a very rare occurrence." The individual who was mugged, however, has been sensitized by his or her personal experience, and will continue to be what the neighbors may consider "overly" cautious.

In the same way, a woman who has had personal experience with breast cancer is more sensitive to the disease. She is not acting irrationally, is not a hypochondriac, and does not have "cancer phobia." Instead, she is responding in a rational manner to her own life experience. One of the goals of Breast Cancer Risk Analysis is to help each woman reach an understanding and acceptance of her level of concern, so she can choose the type of breast health care that will give her the most comfort and safety.

When a Mother Has Breast Cancer

Over the years, I have seen hundreds of women whose mothers had breast cancer. Some were children when their mothers were affected, and others were grown women. Most of the mothers had mastectomies; a few had no surgery at all. More recently, I have seen women whose mothers had a lumpectomy followed by radiation treatment. In some cases, the mother died of breast cancer, while in others she did not. Virtually all of the women I see whose mothers had breast cancer, regardless of their age or the outcome of their mothers' disease, have been profoundly affected by it. These women may suffer from fear, uncertainty, lowered self-esteem, guilt, or a hesitancy to establish close relationships with others. They may worry more than others about the loss of a breast, the possibility of sudden illness, or death. Some feel they have experienced greater difficulty in establishing independence from their mothers.

The following sections provide a sampling of the thoughts and emotions daughters of breast cancer patients have shared with me, and are in no way intended to be comprehensive. From this brief survey, I hope to provide an understanding of the range and depth of the social effects (which could also be called social risks) that may be produced by a mother's breast cancer diagnosis. All family members are affected, of course. Here, however, I focus on the reactions adult daughters have reported to me. For readings of a scientific nature, you might start with the article by Lichtman et al. (1984) which explores relationships between mothers and children following the mother's diagnosis of breast cancer. Preliminary studies on the reactions of daughters are also reported in Kelly (1980) and are being further studied (Wendy Schain and David Wellisch, telephone conversation, 1990).

Lasting Effects

Many daughters have vivid memories of their mother's diagnosis and treatment, even years after the event. For example, Dorothy, a forty-eight-year-old nurse who came to see me fourteen years after her mother's diagnosis, sobbed uncontrollably when beginning to speak about her mother, and then said:

> I'm very sorry. I don't know what's gotten into me. I haven't talked to anyone about this for years. She was so very sick and in so much pain after the surgery. So small, and so little and so helpless lying there in that bed. You know, when you see your mother like that, it tears you apart inside. She's been through so much in her life, why this?

I find that many daughters, like Dorothy, have had little or no opportunity to speak to others about their mothers' breast cancer, and to evaluate its meaning in their lives. Many are surprised by the intensity of their feelings and the new insights they achieve while discussing this experience in depth for the first time.

Some daughters feel that the lack of attention from and guidance by their mothers during the time she was ill helped to produce significant, unfortunate changes in the direction of their lives. Molly, for example, a resigned woman of fifty-three whose conversation was punctuated with sighs, was a young woman in college in another state when her mother was diagnosed. She remembers:

> The operation was very painful and the scar was hideous. It was difficult to simulate normal appearance. I was going back and forth, but it was hard for my family to pay my airfare. I couldn't stand to stay there and watch her like that. Mother hated for me to be there and wanted for me to be there at the same time. Our family situation deteriorated. All of the children married people we wouldn't have otherwise. We all got away from home in the only acceptable way.

For some daughters, the experience with their mothers was so upsetting that their religious faith has been shaken. It is difficult for these women to understand why their mothers were so ill and had so much pain. As one deeply religious daughter said:

> I do believe in God. You have to, you know. I feel that people die when God wants to take them from this life. But sometimes you see the really good people dying and the Mafia people still living and you wonder why. But I suppose each one of us is more ready to meet God when we go. Who would know why God took her at that time?

Following their mothers' diagnoses, some daughters said they felt deprived of the attention they had previously received and taken for granted. Instead of being interested in details of their daughters' lives as they used to, mothers focused more on the pain and fear in their own lives. As a result, daughters sometimes felt they lost their mother before death. This sense of loss was sometimes accompanied by a painful and frightening disorientation. As a consequence, some daughters say they have difficulty experiencing closeness:

> I still think I have problems getting really close to somebody. I have difficulty trusting people. In fact, I told my husband several times, I realize it's very childish, but I carry this feeling that if you really love something, it's going to die. That's the way I feel. Intellectually, I know that's not true. But I've had to really work at having a close personal relationship with anybody.

Learning Mother Has Breast Cancer

Women often tell me they were shocked to learn of their mothers' breast cancer diagnosis. Helen, at the age of thirty-two, fainted when the doctor emerged from the operating room to give the assembled family the diagnosis. Polly, then in her early twenties, was so sure her mother's lump would not be malignant, she arrived at the hospital after the mastectomy was over. Following the initial shock, many daughters become frightened for themselves as well as for their mothers. Anne, a nurse who was working with cancer patients at the time of her mother's diagnosis, said she "went to pieces" but still insisted on teaching her sister breast self-examination techniques the very day her mother was diagnosed. Other daughters quickly called their doctor for a breast examination.

Some daughters became so concerned about their own risk that they ignored their mother in the weeks or months that followed. Sally, a thirty-four-year-old housewife with two very young children, didn't visit her mother for over a year following the diagnosis. She says she now feels terrible about neglecting her mother, but also realizes:

> I was so scared for myself and hurt so much for her, I couldn't bear to be that close. I think she understood, because she didn't encourage me to come till I had it all sorted out.

Following the diagnosis, some daughters had difficulty functioning. Francie, now forty-five, recalls when her mother was ill twenty-five years ago:

> It really shook me up. For the first time in my life I didn't quite know where I was going. I've always been very well directed, know just what I want, and I go and get it. This shook me up real badly.

Daughters who were children or teenagers at the time of their mother's breast cancer diagnosis were not always told about it. In some cases a daughter was aware her mother was ill, but had no idea a mastectomy had been performed, that she had breast cancer, or even was facing a serious illness. Daughters who were teenagers or young adults at the time of their mothers' diagnosis were frequently so involved with school, first jobs, boyfriends, or marriage plans that they tended to accept family reassurances about their mothers' health. For example, Ruth's mother became progressively weaker and was confined to a wheelchair. The children were told their mother had arthritis. It was only in retrospect, or when their mothers' condition worsened, that many women say they realized their mother had breast cancer and was seriously ill.

Some families hid the nature and seriousness of the mothers' illness to such an extent that daughters were completely unprepared for a worsening condition or death. When these daughters finally realized their mother had been dealing with a life-threatening illness for years, they felt tremendously guilty for not helping more around the house, for not giving their mother more emotional support, or for not being more affectionate. Harriet, now aged thirty-six, was completely unprepared at age seventeen when her mother died:

> I was at home, but my father didn't even tell me that she had breast cancer or anything. I asked her once if she had cancer and she said no. They were trying to protect me, but I was old enough that I should have known.

She still has nightmares about the day her mother unexpectedly died.

Daughters who were children and were not told of the diagnosis or severity of their mother's illness sometimes resented others who tried to help. For example, Marie remembers her grandmother coming to take care of her and her brothers and sisters when her mother was quite ill:

> I know I hated my grandmother. She took my mother's place and she was not my mother. I remember saying things like that to her.

In some cases, daughters were so upset that they made normal family interactions almost impossible. Their delinquency ranged from skipping school, to stealing, to starting fires. Some, like Linda, railed against their fathers:

> I was so snotty and I wasn't a nice girl. I hated my father. I hated him for years. He never would tell me that she was going to die and he always acted like everything was going to be all right. And I knew it wouldn't. I guess for his inability to make things O.K., he wasn't a good daddy.

Without realizing it, these daughters may judge their behavior as children or adolescents by adult standards. It can be quite useful for them to realize that they were children then, reacting to stresses and changes as children do. To my amazement, very few of the daughters had ever spoken to a therapist or even a family friend to begin to put these experiences into perspective.

By learning about women's reactions to their mothers' breast cancer, health professionals may be better prepared to help patients deal with issues from the past that prevent them either from hearing and understanding new information or from following reasonable breast health practices. In some cases, a woman's realization that her childhood reactions were normal will be sufficient. In others, help from a mental health professional may be necessary.

Guilt

The daughters I see are like other daughters—they compare themselves to their mothers, love their mothers, and try to live up to the image of what they think their mothers would want them to be. They also criticize their mothers, rail against their mothers' way of life, and stoutly declare that they are their own women and no longer dependent on mother. The daughters of breast cancer patients are not immune to the anger or guilt that arises in other families; indeed, they might have particularly burdensome feelings of guilt as a result of their mothers' illness. As discussed earlier, some adult daughters feel guilty for not giving their mothers more emotional or physical help when they were children. The realization that they were unhappy children with big emotional problems helps some to deal with their feelings of guilt. Others come to realize that their guilt feelings are heightened when they judge the children they were by adult standards.

Daughters who were teenagers or adults when their mother was diagnosed may feel guilty about the lack of attention they paid to their mothers' illness. Many say they carefully avoided mentioning breast cancer or illness for fear their mother would think they were prying or overstepping their role in the mother-daughter relationship. In retrospect, they worry that they didn't inquire enough, leaving their mothers to feel alone and unloved.

Some daughters blame themselves for directly causing their mothers' breast cancer. They fear that their difficult behavior led to aggravation, which in turn caused the disease. They may even wonder, as Gail does, if their birth caused the breast cancer:

> I was the last of six born very close together. It can't be good to have that many children all at once.

Others are convinced that a past action on their part helped to cause the breast cancer. For example, one woman left her infant son in her mother's care several extra hours one day.

During this time, he kicked her mother in the breast. She was convinced that her mother's breast cancer, which developed fifteen years later, was due to this kick—and her own tardy behavior.

Risk to Self

In assessing their own risk of breast cancer daughters may compare themselves to their mothers and conclude that with increased similarities in personality or physique their own risk is increased. As one thoughtful health professional, whose mother was affected twenty years previously, said:

> My chances are very good that I'm going to have a mastectomy some time in my life. And I don't know how I'm going to feel about it. I won't be shocked if I have a mastectomy. But how I will deal with it emotionally—whether I will cry myself to sleep or go through all these emotions I've seen women go through—I don't know. I'm only human. I don't know whether I can put on a front or not.

Even this well-informed individual, who was intellectually aware of breast conserving treatments for breast cancer, automatically assumed that if she were to be diagnosed with the disease, the treatment would be the same as her mother's—mastectomy and arm edema.

Those whose mothers have died often make the further unfortunate assumption that they will also die of breast cancer. As noted earlier, adult women may realize intellectually that current early detection of breast cancer improves the prognosis for many women, but fail to apply this information to their own situation. As children, this assumption may also be present. Donna, who was twelve when her mother died, said:

> I remember thinking during those weeks something like, "Well, this means that I will have to die of breast cancer."

> I was very clear about that. "But that won't be for a long time." So I kind of postponed it. But I guess I still believe it.

Breast Cancer Risk Analysis can help patients realize that they are not doomed to follow the types of treatment nor the outcomes suffered by their relatives.

It's not surprising, really, that many women whose mothers had breast cancer are concerned that they, too, will get the disease. Many say they suffer a constant undercurrent of worry, a feeling of anxiety that can surface during times of stress. As Laurie put it:

> When my sister and I get sick, we worry. I don't think I have cancer, but if I have even a cold, there's a taste of anxiety underneath.

As women approach the age at which their mothers were diagnosed, their anxiety often increases. As they pass that age, they may begin to feel they are sufficiently different from their mothers and might not get breast cancer after all. Unfortunately, some become overconfident, feeling that all danger has passed, and so may fail to maintain adequate breast health care. Those who believe they differ from their mothers may erroneously think their risks are diminished:

> Well, with it inherited, I assume that I could get it. But I'm not like my mother in build or anything else, like disposition. I'm more like an aunt on my father's side of the family. So I assume that maybe I have more of her genes than I do of my mother's.

In an attempt to avoid breast cancer, daughters may take active steps to try to become different from their mothers—often not realizing how difficult it would be to effect a significant change. For example, Sylvia is a forty-year-old physician, dedicated to her profession. She says her mother is a hypochondriac who suffered from many ailments, real and imagined. Sylvia maintains that she became a physician to get as far away as possible from her mother's concerns, and believes she has. But Sylvia, like many daughters, is not really as different from her mother as she thinks she is. Both she and her mother spend much of their time focused on disease—the mother on her own and Sylvia on that of others. Other lifestyle differences daughters often cite include more activity, less obesity, greater assertiveness, and being more in control of their own destinies than were their mothers.

Daughters who try to be different from their mothers are often conflicted. If they accept their resemblance to their mothers, they may worry that this resemblance will increase their risk of breast cancer. If, in an effort to lower their breast cancer risk, they deny their similarity to their mothers, or focus on differences in personality or lifestyle, they may find themselves alienated not just from their mothers, but from important facets of themselves.

A Service for Families

Women are often helped by knowing more about the results of scientific studies pertaining to risks of breast cancer associated with factors such as personality and stress (see Chapter 4), and family history (see Chapter 6). They are eager to learn about new techniques that make early detection of breast cancer more feasible (see Chapter 7), and about how others in a similar situation have reacted. Many daughters who were children or teenagers when their mothers had breast cancer are amazed to learn that other daughters have experienced similar feelings and reactions. Whatever their reactions, most assumed they were not normal and would have been greatly helped by having a trained professional to speak to about their fears and concerns, right from the time their mother was diagnosed.

I have great respect for the unique sorrows and cares expressed by daughters of breast cancer patients—and for their strengths. Unfortunately, many do not realize how heroic and helpful they were and continue to be. Many are surprised to learn that their reactions, fears, and uncertainties are not due to an inherent weakness in themselves, but are shared by many other daughters and are normal responses to a mother's breast cancer diagnosis. In our society, classes are offered if a woman wants to learn how to play the piano, ski, invest in real estate, or have a baby. However, when an individual or her relative has a breast problem or breast cancer, instruction about the issues she and relatives can expect to face are generally not available.

I would like to see the development and spread of programs similar to those now offered to daughters and other relatives of breast cancer patients as part of Breast Cancer Risk Analysis Services (see Appendix A). At the time of a breast cancer diagnosis, families could be helped in dealing with the fears and uncertainties that face them, if they were informed about the feelings and experiences others have had in similar situations: young girls then would not be left to wonder alone if they will also get breast cancer one day; spouses and other family members would be less uncertain about how to talk to their loved one with breast cancer; parents would not have to wrestle alone with how much and when to tell the children. Instead, the whole family would receive the necessary support and information to help them better deal with the situation in which they so suddenly find themselves.

SUMMARY

Daughters of women with breast cancer have unique experiences which often shape their views of the world, of themselves, and of their breast cancer risk. Although experiences vary, some common threads emerge. These include feelings of shock and grief when a mother is first diagnosed. Many feel their lives were changed irrevocably by the illness, leaving them with increased insecurities and with increased concerns about illness in general. Many daughters benefit from an opportunity to speak to a trained mental health professional to work through the stresses and concerns that often follow their mothers' breast cancer diagnosis. Daughters and their families need better access to medical, scientific, and social information from the time of the breast cancer diagnosis in the family. By examining patients' beliefs about the causes of breast cancer, as well as their reactions to breast cancer or a breast concern, health professionals can attain a better understanding of the type of information each patient needs.

2

Evaluation of Breast Cancer Risk

As I escorted Marilou into my office, I noticed that she was tense and had started to tremble. Shortly after we sat down, she began to cry. Apologizing for not being able to control her tears, she said, "I'm so embarrassed, you must think I'm a big baby. It's just that my doctor says I'm at very high risk of breast cancer. He says I'm a walking time bomb that could go off at any minute." As we talked, Marilou was surprised to learn that many, many women have been told or feel that it's not a matter of *whether* they will develop breast cancer, but *when*. Like Marilou, large numbers of women are told their risk is increased or high, but receive no specific numbers or formal risk analysis. Instead they are sternly admonished to be careful, or even to have their breasts removed due to what has been called a high or significant risk. Such imprecise terminology can be greatly misleading and cause needless anxiety to patients.

A woman concerned about her breast cancer risk may interpret increased risk as the inevitability of breast cancer or may assume a diagnosis of breast cancer means she will lose her breast and die. For reasons discussed earlier, she may not appreciate that with early detection and today's treatments, the loss of a breast and a grim prognosis are not a foregone conclusion for her. Even well-educated women may lack access to this new information or may fail to appreciate its significance to their own lives.

Many women believe their risk of breast cancer to be much higher than it actually is. For example, Marilou was very concerned about her breast cancer risk, estimating it to be 85 percent or higher because she had had a breast biopsy five years previously and was nulliparous, and her mother had breast cancer. My formal analysis showed that Marilou's lifetime risk of breast cancer was about 20 percent, with a risk in the next 10 years of less than 1 percent a year—far lower than the 85 percent risk she believed at the time of our first meeting. Initially, of course, I didn't have enough information to analyze her breast cancer risk, and so I explained that I would like to proceed in a scientific manner to determine her risk more precisely. To do so, I would need specific information about her breast biopsy and family history.

Risk Analysis Procedure

First, Marilou and I reviewed a questionnaire she had completed before the first visit. From this, I learned about her own past medical history and her family history of breast and other cancers. I also learned that she had had two previous mammograms and a breast biopsy.

Marilou was surprised when I asked for permission to order her mammograms and biopsy slides for review. I told her that since she had come for a thorough analysis, I would feel more confident if we received a second opinion regarding these materials from physicians who specialize in breast health care. The pathology review would enable me to give her more precise risk information, based on the specific type of benign breast disease present (see Chapter 3), while a review of her mammograms would provide confirmation of the original reading and a check on the previous institution's quality. With this information she would be better prepared to work with her physician to plan a breast health program suited to her needs.

In reviewing Marilou's family history, I learned that her

Figure 2-1. Incidence of Breast Cancer in U.S. Women by Age

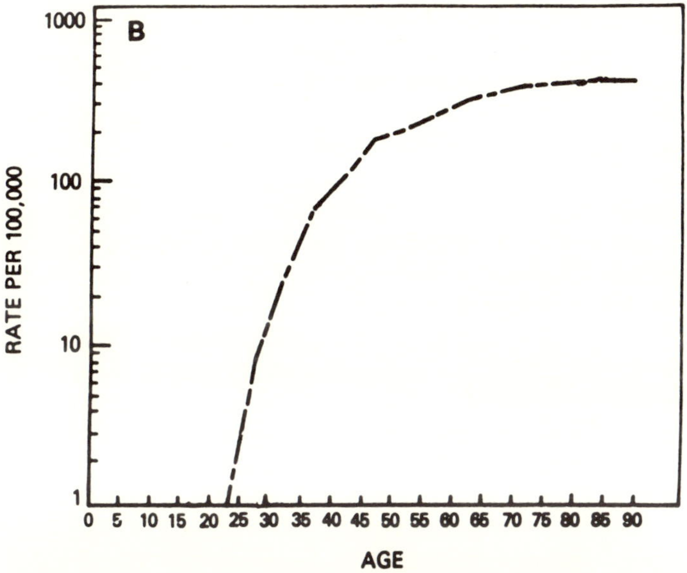

Source: Horm, J. W., A. J. Asire, J. L. Young et al., eds., 1984, *SEER Program: Cancer Incidence and Mortality in the United States 1973–1981*. DHHS Publication No. (NIH) 85-1837. Bethesda, Md.: NIH.

mother and maternal grandmother had had breast cancer and that her maternal aunt had had breast surgery of some sort. Her mother's, grandmother's, and aunt's pathology reports were also ordered (see Chapter 6).

Average Woman's Breast Cancer Risk

During our first visit, I began to give Marilou background information about breast cancer risk—and some guidance about how to evaluate risk figures and scientific studies. First I showed her a graph on which it could be seen that in the United States, as women get older, their risk of breast cancer increases (see Figure 2-1).

I then noted that speaking about risk without specifying time is as uninformative as talking about speed without indicating time. For example, if one wants to know how fast an object is moving, it is not sufficient to say sixty miles; in addition, one needs to know whether it is moving at sixty miles per hour, per minute, or per second. Similarly, when discussing breast cancer risk, one needs to know whether a risk pertains to one year, ten years, or one hundred ten years. Many health professionals are aware of American Cancer Society figures which showed that in 1988, the average white woman in the United States had a 10 percent risk of developing breast cancer. It is important to realize that this 10 percent figure is the lifetime cumulative risk for all white women—that is, the risk from birth up to about age one hundred ten (Herbert Seidman, letter to author, 1987).

The concept of cumulative risk might be better understood if it is supposed that a woman must cross a busy street once a year, every year of her life. Each time she crosses the street, there is a chance she will be hit by a car. A young woman's lifetime risk of being hit is higher than that of an older woman's, because the younger woman probably has more years ahead of her, and so over the years will cross the street more times than will the older one. Alternatively, the older woman has successfully crossed the street without incident many years, and so is no longer at risk for the street crossings that have passed. Further, if we assume a younger woman is more agile and has better eyesight than an older woman, the younger will be at less risk of being hit during one trip across the street. So, although the lifetime risk of breast cancer is higher for younger women than for older, for a given year (a single street crossing), the risk is lower for the younger than the older.

According to American Cancer Society calculations, in 1987 the average white woman's risk was about 2 percent from birth to age fifty and 6 percent from birth to age seventy (Herbert Seidman, letter, 1987). Only if a woman were to live to age one hundred ten would her risk be 10 percent. The 10 percent cumulative risk is the sum of women's risks from

Table 2-1. Selected Age-Specific Risks of Breast Cancer, U.S. Black Women, 1987

Age	Risk of Developing	Risk of Dying
35–45	0.9%	0.2%
35–55	2.4	0.6
35–110	8.1	2.9
50–60	1.8	0.3
50–70	3.6	0.9
50–110	7.0	2.0
65–75	2.4	0.3
65–85	4.5	0.7
65–110	5.3	1.1

Source: Herbert Seidman, letter to author, 1987.

ages twenty to thirty, plus the risks from thirty to forty and so on, up to age one hundred ten. The average black woman's risk was a little lower—about 8 percent to age one hundred ten—but is rapidly approaching that of white women, so the figures for white women are used here. (However, please see Table 2-1 for the 1987 age-specific risks for blacks.) Asian women have a lower risk than blacks or whites. For example, one study found that women of Japanese ancestry had a risk about half that of white women (Nomura et al. 1984).

Table 2-2 shows the average white woman's risk of breast cancer by age. As you can see, from thirty-five to forty-five the risk is 1 percent, and from thirty-five to fifty-five it is higher—about 2.5 percent—because more years are involved. A thirty-five-year-old woman has a lifetime risk of 10 percent. Now consider the risk for a fifty-year-old woman. From fifty to sixty her risk is 2 percent, and from fifty to seventy about 5 percent. At age fifty, her lifetime risk has dropped from 10 percent to 8.8 percent. By successfully reaching age fifty without a diagnosis of breast cancer, she leaves behind the risk up to age fifty, and faces the risk after fifty only. (Due to statistical complexities and rounding-

Table 2-2. Selected Age-Specific Risks of Breast Cancer, U.S. White Women, 1987

Age	Risk of Developing	Risk of Dying
35–45	1.0%	0.1%
35–55	2.6	0.1
35–110	10.0	3.4
50–60	2.0	0.3
50–70	4.7	1.0
50–110	8.8	2.5
65–75	3.0	0.4
65–85	5.3	0.9
65–110	6.3	1.3

Source: Herbert Seidman, letter to author, 1987.

off, one cannot simply subtract 2 percent from 10 percent, leaving a fifty-year-old woman with an 8 percent risk.)

Patients are generally quite surprised by the difference between cumulative and age-specific risks. Marilou, for example, explained that she would look around at meetings and assume that one out of the ten women present would develop breast cancer in the next few years. "After all," she said, "I keep hearing that the risk of breast cancer to young women is increasing. In five years, it sometimes seems most of us will have it." Marilou was intrigued when she learned that the numerical increase in risk to young women is small, and may be due in part to the more frequent use of early detection techniques by this group.

I showed Marilou Table 2-3, which compares the risk of breast cancer in white women in 1987 and 1978. For women aged thirty-five to forty-five, and those aged fifty to sixty, the risk increased by only 0.2 percent from 1978 to 1987. Even among those aged sixty-five to seventy-five, the increase in breast cancer risk was less than 1 percent. These risks tell only part of the story, so I also showed Marilou Table 2-4, which compares the death rate due to breast cancer in 1987

Table 2-3. Age-Specific Risks of Developing Breast Cancer, U.S. White Women, 1987 and 1978

	Risk	
Age	*1987*	*1978*
20–30	0.1%	0.1%
20–40	0.5	0.4
20–110	10.0	7.9
35–45	1.0	0.8
35–55	2.6	2.3
35–110	10.0	7.9
50–60	2.0	1.8
50–70	4.7	3.7
50–110	8.8	6.7
65–75	3.0	2.2
65–85	5.3	4.0
65–110	6.3	4.5

Sources: Herbert Seidman, letter to author, 1987; Herbert Seidman. 1978. "Screening for Breast Cancer in Younger Women: Life Expectancy Gains and Losses," *Ca—A Cancer Journal for Clinicians* 27:66–87.

and 1978. During these nine years the rate dropped from 0.2 percent to 0.1 percent for those thirty-five to forty-five, stayed the same for the fifty- to sixty-year-olds, and increased only 0.1 percent for women aged sixty-five to seventy-five. In other words, even with an increase in the incidence, the death rate either declined or was less than the increase in incidence.

Evaluating Studies

The following guidelines are useful in analyzing studies and helping patients understand why some studies are more reliable than others.

Table 2-4. Age-Specific Risks of Dying of Breast Cancer, U.S. White Women, 1987 and 1978

	Risk	
Age	*1987*	*1978*
20–30	0.01%	0.01%
20–40	0.1	0.1
20–110	3.5	3.1
35–45	0.1	0.2
35–55	0.1	0.6
35–110	3.4	3.0
50–60	0.3	0.3
50–70	1.0	0.9
50–110	2.5	2.2
65–75	0.4	0.3
65–85	0.9	0.8
65–110	1.3	1.1

Sources: Herbert Seidman, letter to author, 1987; Herbert Seidman. 1978. "Screening for Breast Cancer in Younger Women: Life Expectancy Gains and Losses," *Ca—A Cancer Journal for Clinicians* 27:66–87.

Time Frame

The above discussion on differences between lifetime risk and age-specific risk demonstrates how misleading it can be to discuss risk without specifying the time over which the risk applies or the age of the individual.

Sample Size

There is no hard and fast rule about the number of individuals needed in a study to produce accurate results. Usually, the larger the number, the more exact the results, if the study has been properly designed in other ways. A group of fewer than fifty subjects is rarely convincing or definitive.

Definition of a Risk Factor

A risk factor is any presumed agent, genetic or environmental, that is thought to affect risk. The definition of a risk factor is of great importance in assessing the clinical application of any study's finding. For example, a study of benign breast disease as a risk factor for breast cancer without further clarification of the term is not likely to provide useful information to an individual patient because benign breast disease is a catchall category that includes many different cell types. In the same way, a study on childhood diseases would not be as useful as one on measles or chicken pox.

Retrospective and Prospective Studies

Studies are organized in two main ways; either they start with a group of affected individuals and look back in their medical and family histories to see which factors are associated with the disease (retrospective), or they start with a group of unaffected individuals and follow them over a period of time to determine who becomes affected (prospective). It is more difficult to identify potential biases in the selection of study and control groups in a retrospective than in a prospective study. For example, we don't know all of the factors affecting breast cancer risk, so it can be difficult to know which criteria to use in selecting a control group for a retrospective study. In a prospective study, the incidence of the disease in question can be directly compared in the study and control groups. However, in a retrospective study, an estimate of the risk is obtained, as explained below in the discussion of relative risk.

Selection of a Control Group

In a prospective epidemiologic study on breast cancer risk, those women with a given risk factor, such as benign breast disease (the study group), and those women without the risk factor (the control group), are compared with regard to the development of breast cancer. Usually, the risk of breast cancer in the control group is assigned the number 1.0.

The control group is generally chosen to be as similar as possible to the study group in factors such as age, ethnicity, and socio-economic status. Often, the control group is selected from the general population or from a hospital population. Obviously, no control group is perfect, since we do not as yet know many of the factors influencing breast cancer risk. Because breast cancer can exist undetected for years, one expects to find a higher rate of breast cancer in a study group if it has access to more regular medical examinations (for example, women using oral contraceptives) than a control group of nonusers drawn from the general population. This bias is elegantly discussed by Feinstein (1988), who also notes that hospital controls have their own problems, since different institutions admit different types of patients.

Relative Risk

This is a way to compare differences in risk between the study and control groups. For example, the relative risks in the study group might be reported as 1.2 or 0.6. This means that the study group is 1.2 times more likely or 0.6 times likely (that is, less likely) than the control group to be diagnosed with breast cancer (or any other trait being studied). In some cases, the control group will have a higher risk than average and in some cases, lower, depending on its composition—age and other risk factors—that influences the overall risk to the control group. In a well-designed study, these variations can be minimized by statistically adjusting for differences between the study and control groups.

One cannot generally arrive at an estimate of the percent risk (which many patients consider the "real" risk) by multiplying a relative risk (such as 1.2 or 0.6) by the average woman's lifetime risk of breast cancer. Relative risk represents the specific rate of disease in a given study group compared to its control group. Unless one has access to the data collected during the study, it is usually impossible to convert a relative risk to a percentage. A relative risk multiplied by the average woman's lifetime risk does not produce an accurate percent because the average risk is obtained by considering all women—those with and those without the risk factor in question. Also, the lifetime risk is the risk to age one hundred ten. Since few if any of the women in most studies are over eighty, their cumulative risk is less than 10 percent. If one were to use the lifetime risk, it would apply only to women who lived to be over one hundred.

Significant Difference

Just as a perfectly sound penny can be flipped three times and three times come up heads due to chance alone, so two groups can differ in breast cancer rates due to chance alone. Statisticians use tests of significance to determine how likely it is that differences between two groups are due to chance (and therefore not to the factor being studied). Most tests use a cutoff of 0.05 or 5 percent. That is, a difference is said to be significant when it is large enough to occur by chance alone 5 percent of the time or less. If the differences between the two groups were due to chance, one would obtain a significant finding 5 percent of the time.

Because of the factor of chance, I feel more confident in study findings when several research groups obtain similar results. Remember, however, that a statistically significant difference is not necessarily one that is large. It refers only to a difference that is not likely (with a 95 percent probability) to be due to chance alone.

Confidence Intervals

Ninety-five percent confidence intervals specify the range within which the true value of the relative risk will be found, 95 percent of the time, if the study were repeated many times. In other words, the confidence interval tells how much uncertainty there is about the true value of the relative risk.

A narrow confidence interval suggests a precise estimate of relative risk, whereas a wide confidence interval suggests findings that one should interpret cautiously until they are confirmed by others, preferably using larger numbers of individuals in the study and control groups. Generally speaking, the smaller the numbers in the groups being studied, the larger the confidence interval—and the more likely the difference between the groups is due to chance. Confidence intervals, which are usually placed in parentheses after the relative risk, are used to judge whether a significant difference is present. If the relative risk 1.0 is included in the confidence interval, this suggests that there could be no appreciable or significant difference between the groups being studied. That is, the observed difference could be due to chance.

Association or Cause?

Epidemiological studies usually measure whether a group with a given factor is or is not at increased risk, compared to a group that lacks the given factor, but is similar in other ways, such as ethnicity, age, socioeconomic status, and other known risk factors. In other words, these are typically studies of association, not cause. The factor associated with increased risk could be a causative agent, but cause cannot be proven in studies of this type. Prospective studies offer more conclusive evidence of causation than do those that are retrospective.

Remember, even if a high association is found between a factor and breast cancer risk, this does not necessarily mean the factor caused the disease. For example, individuals at increased risk of lung cancer may be statistically more likely to carry matches. Similarly, countries with more television sets have a higher incidence of breast cancer than do those with fewer. Matches are not thought to cause lung cancer, nor are television sets thought to be responsible for the increased breast cancer incidence. Instead, matches and television sets are associated with, or are more likely to be present when other factors, which do increase risk are also present.

When new risk factors are identified in research, it is impossible to know at first whether the association is biologically causal or not. The association may prove to be linked to a related factor which is itself a causal factor. For example, studies some years ago found increased parity (having borne children) was associated with decreased breast cancer risk. Later it became apparent that women with increased parity generally gave birth to their first child at a younger age than those with lower parity. Younger age at first birth is now thought by many to be responsible for the decrease in risk, not the number of children. Increased parity, like television sets, acted as a marker for decreased risk, but was not itself the risk factor.

The tentativeness of epidemiological research findings may be obscured by conventional terms used in describing them. For example, when discussing study results, scientists often say a study "found" or "showed" an increase or decrease in risk. It is critical to remember that this is a shorthand method for saying "found an association" between a given factor and breast cancer risk. The association may or may not prove to be a causal factor.

Publication Bias

Given the rigors of bringing a study through the publication process, it is not surprising that a study in which no association is found between a given factor and breast cancer risk is more likely to remain in the investigator's filing cabinet than is a study in which an association is found. For this reason, more studies showing a positive association than not are likely to be published (Cook 1989). Therefore, one cannot simply compare the number of studies which do and do not find an association with a given risk factor to determine how seriously to consider the factor. Instead, it is important to assess the overall weight of evidence that includes the types and sizes of studies in which associations are reported.

Percent Increases in Risk

Many patients are frightened by terms such as a 50 percent or 100 percent increase in risk. And yet even a 100 percent increase can result in a very small numerical difference. For example, in the United States, the average white woman's risk of breast cancer from ages thirty to forty was about 1 percent in 1987. A 50 percent increase in this age group's risk is 1 percent plus 0.5 percent or 1.5 percent. A 100 percent increase in risk is 1 percent plus 1 percent or 2 percent—hardly as scary as the terms 50 percent and 100 percent imply. For this reason, it is important to learn the size of the original risk before assuming that an increase is large.

Differences in Techniques or Regimens Over Time

Research literature can be difficult to assess when published findings are based on outdated practices or technology. Two examples immediately come to mind: mammography and hormone replacement therapy. Recent studies on the fifteen- or twenty-year effects on breast cancer death rates of early detection by mammography must rely on mammograms taken fifteen to twenty years ago. In this time, mammogram technology has greatly improved, so studies with long-term follow-up apply to outmoded techniques, not to today's improved technology. Hormone replacement therapy has also changed in the last twenty years. These days, physicians generally use far lower doses than in the past, and include hormones other than estrogen in their regimen (see Chapter 5). In assessing the relevance of studies to your patients, it is important to be clear about the extent to which the techniques and practices studied differ from those of today.

Life Table Analysis

The accurate determination of risk over time may necessitate more than the calculation of percentage affected. When simple percentages are used, later cases of affected individuals carry more weight than those detected earlier, because the size of the group at risk diminishes over time. For calculation purposes, individuals are removed from study and control groups when they are diagnosed with the disease being studied or die of any cause. For example, if a study group initially consists of fifty women, at the end of thirty-five years, it may contain only ten. The diagnosis of a single case at the beginning of a study will produce a very different percent from one at the end (one out of fifty is 2 percent at the beginning while one out of ten is 10 percent at the end). For this reason, more complex calculations are used that take the decreasing denominator into account and are called life table analysis. (For a more thorough presentation of this methodology, see Lilienfeld 1976; Hill 1971.)

I will be discussing these and other statistical aspects of studies as each specific risk factor is considered. I mention them here to emphasize that current epidemiological methods that rely on observation of disease occurrence or diagnosis in human study groups cannot determine cause and effect relationships in the scientific manner used in a laboratory (Feinstein 1988). Observational studies reveal statistical associations and help in the inference rather than in the proof of causality.

SUMMARY

Most women are surprised to learn that their risk of breast cancer is lower than they had expected. To accurately determine a woman's risk, it is necessary to examine her own and her relatives' medical records. Generalizations about risk can be misleading and frightening, so records are well worth obtaining.

In evaluating studies, it is important to look at the size of the groups compared, how carefully risk factors are defined, and to be aware that a significant percent increase in risk, or even a 100 percent increase in risk, does not necessarily mean a large numerical increase. Even when a significant difference in risk is found between a study and control group, various methodological issues must be weighed before a given association (not cause) can be accepted as clinically useful. In determining the relevance of a given risk factor to patients, the bulk of the evidence, as set forth in several studies, must be carefully weighed.

3

Benign Breast "Disease" and Non-invasive "Cancers"

Breast changes do not lead inexorably to breast cancer. This chapter discusses and distinguishes between different types of breast changes that are not breast cancer.

Benign Breast "Disease"

Benign breast disease (also called cystic breasts, fibrocystic breast disease, lumpy breasts, and so forth) is a catchall term that includes many different processes. Most women, sometime during their lives, will notice a lumpiness or nodularity of the breasts. Many experience an increase in breast nodularity or a feeling of breast fullness just prior to menstruation, with symptoms subsiding afterward. In this chapter, for want of a better term, I refer to all breast lumps, cysts, and areas of thickening as benign breast disease. Many experts decry the use of the term "disease" for so prevalent a condition. For example, a pathologist colleague notes that even when breast changes are accompanied by pain or feelings of fullness, these are natural changes and do not represent actual disease but only exaggerated physiologic reaction.

Benign breast disease and breast cancer typically arise in small clusters of interconnected milk ducts called the termi-

Figure 3-1. Progression of Cell Changes in Breast Duct

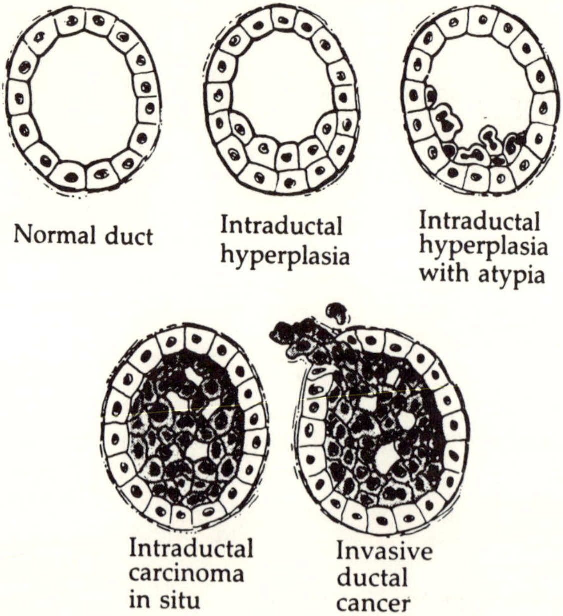

Source: Susan M. Love, M.D., *Dr. Susan Love's Breast Book*, © 1990, by Susan M. Love, M.D. Illustrations by Marcia Williams. Figures 14-2 and 14-3. Reprinted with permission of Addison-Wesley Publishing Co., Inc., Reading, Massachusetts.

nal ducto-lobular units. Figure 3-1 shows a progression of cell changes in the duct lining, from normal to hyperplasia without atypia, to hyperplasia with atypia, to in situ breast cancer, to invasive breast cancer.

Only following a breast biopsy is it possible to determine the type of benign breast disease (if any) that is present. These days, of course, most breast biopsies are performed under local anesthesia and are excisional, not incisional. At the time of surgery, tissue may be frozen to enable a quick pathologic diagnosis (frozen section). This is not generally recommended in current practice, however, since the most accurate findings are available only when the permanent sections have been analyzed, which may take several days.

Until just a few years ago, most studies on benign breast disease reported that all women with this condition were at increased risk of breast cancer. However, these studies did not take the heterogeneity of benign breast disease into account, and so considered as a group all women with any form of benign breast disease. By combining women who were and were not at increased risk of breast cancer, the group as a whole was found to have a somewhat higher than average breast cancer risk. To help my patients grasp the concept of heterogeneity, I ask them to imagine a gallon container 95 percent filled with clear water. In this case, clear water represents the vast majority of women who have a type of benign breast disease that does not increase breast cancer risk. To this clear water, they add 5 percent of a gallon of red ink, which represents the small proportion of women who have a type of benign breast disease that is associated with increased breast cancer risk. Now the whole gallon looks pink, when in actuality, two different populations are present, the one at increased risk (red ink) and the other not (clear water).

Several excellent studies have now shown that women with benign breast disease are a heterogeneous group. Those who had atypical cells or atypia were found to be at significantly increased risk of breast cancer, while those with other types of benign breast disease were not. Atypia refers to the size and shape of the cell and its nucleus, as well as the kind of intercellular arrangements found. (I remind patients that only a pathologist, looking at permanent sections of tissue under a microscope, can distinguish between different types of benign breast disease.) There are many types of benign breast disease, but a significant increase in risk is primarily confined to women found to have atypia. From 3 percent to 5 percent of benign breast disease biopsies are found to have atypical cells.

There are two types of atypia: atypical ductal hyperplasia (ADH) and atypical lobular hyperplasia (ALH). Hyperplasia

Table 3-1. Risk of Breast Cancer to Women with Atypical Ductal Hyperplasia

Years after Biopsy	Risk in Those Years*
0–5	5%
6–10	5
11–15	2

*122 women at risk; none had affected mother or sister; 11 developed breast cancer over 20 years. Risks calculated using life table analysis.
Source: Adapted from D. L. Page, et al., 1985. "Atypical Hyperplastic Lesions of the Female Breast," *Cancer* 55:2698–2708. Reprinted by permission of the copyright owner, *Cancer* and J. B. Lippincott Company.

Table 3-2. Risk of Breast Cancer to Women with Atypical Lobular Hyperplasia

Years after Biopsy	Risk in Those Years*
0–5	1%
6–10	6
11–15	3

*107 women at risk; none had affected mother or sister; 11 developed breast cancer over 20 years. Risks calculated using life table analysis.
Source: Adapted from D. L. Page, et al., 1985. "Atypical Hyperplastic Lesions of the Female Breast," *Cancer* 55:2698–2708. Reprinted by permission of the copyright owner, *Cancer* and J. B. Lippincott Company.

is an abnormal increase in the number of cells. Regardless of type, a finding of atypia is associated with about a 10 percent chance of developing breast cancer over the next ten years (Page et al. 1985). These risks are presented in greater detail in Tables 3-1 and 3-2. The percentages in these tables were obtained by life table analysis. (See Chapter 2 for a brief discussion of this method.)

Table 3-1 considers the first fifteen years following a woman's diagnosis of atypical ductal hyperplasia and demonstrates that in the first ten years, the risk is 1 percent a year to a woman who has no close relative with breast cancer. When that woman has reached the end of the tenth year and does not have breast cancer, the risk over the next five years is 2 percent. Women in the San Francisco Bay area grasp this notion quickly when I compare it with the risk of being injured in an earthquake. Once an earthquake has passed, one cannot be injured by it; an individual remains at risk only of future earthquakes.

Table 3-2 is a summary of the risk of breast cancer following a diagnosis of atypical lobular hyperplasia in women who have no close relative with breast cancer. In this case, the risk over the first five years is 1 percent. From six to ten years, the risk is 6 percent—about 1 percent a year. The risk from eleven to fifteen years is about 2 percent a year. These risks are based on relatively small groups of women, and so should be considered approximations of an individual woman's risk.

The results of the study on atypia provide a good example of how misleading relative risk can be. In this study, women with atypia were found to have a risk of breast cancer three to four times higher than women in the general population in Atlanta who comprised the control group. Moreover, as just discussed above, this turned out to be a risk of about 10 percent in ten years, and 10 percent to 12 percent in fifteen years—not the 30 percent to 40 percent that would be obtained if a three- to four-fold increase in risk were multiplied by the lifetime risk of 10 percent.

Understandably, most women are quite concerned when they learn they have benign breast disease or atypia. Terry is a forty-eight-year-old woman who says her breasts have always been lumpy, leading her to believe her breast cancer risk was high. Her concern increased considerably when she was found to have atypical lobular hyperplasia. She explained:

> When I heard my risk was *significantly* higher, I think I stopped breathing. Then when the doctor said this condition increased my risk to three times that of other women, I got really scared. I was sure I would have breast cancer

before I was fifty-five. I just didn't know how to live with that high a risk.

Terry did not realize that statistically, "significant" means only that the difference between women with and without atypia is greater than a difference expected by chance alone. It is not a description of the importance of the difference or the likelihood that a particular woman will develop breast cancer.

Actually, as the life table analyses in Tables 3-1 and 3-2 show, most women with atypia were never diagnosed with breast cancer. In fact, of those with atypia and no mother or sister with breast cancer, we would expect about 90 percent to be unaffected ten years following their diagnosis of atypia. After learning more about her risk due to atypia, Terry asked what she could do to best protect her health. Some guidelines your patients might find useful are discussed in Chapter 7.

In summary, benign breast disease (fibrocystic disease) is a catchall term which includes a number of microscopically distinct cellular changes in the breast, and can be diagnosed only by a pathologist following a breast biopsy. Recent studies have shown that a minority of women with benign breast disease (those with atypia) are at significantly increased risk of breast cancer. Even among those with atypia, however, most are never diagnosed with breast cancer.

Duct Carcinoma In Situ

Physicians have been aware of invasive breast cancer for thousands of years. However, it was not until the early twentieth century that noninvasive breast cancers were described. There are two types of noninvasive or in situ breast cancers. In this section, I will discuss duct carcinoma in situ (DCIS), which is also called intraductal carcinoma. Lobular carcinoma in situ (LCIS) is discussed below.

Until recently, DCIS was rarely found unless invasive breast cancer was also present. These days, with women having breast biopsies more frequently, with increased use of mammography, and with advances in the quality of mammographic techniques, breast changes are more likely to be diagnosed at an earlier stage, when invasive breast cancer is not present.

DCIS is often, but not always, detected by the presence of calcifications on a mammogram. Calcifications associated with DCIS are generally produced when some of the cells die, producing local changes in the pH. As a result of the change in pH, calcium salts from the blood are deposited in the area of the DCIS. In many cases, when calcifications are removed, no DCIS is found. Calcifications that are grouped and form linear, branching patterns are generally considered sufficiently suspicious of DCIS or invasive disease to warrant a breast biopsy.

DCIS may also be found when no calcifications are present. In most such cases, women are advised to have a mastectomy, since DCIS does not usually form a breast lump and so may not be seen on a mammogram or felt in a breast examination. Some centers offer radiation treatment for DCIS (see Lagios et al. 1989, for a summary). In this section, I discuss DCIS that is associated with calcifications, but where no invasive breast cancer is found. When invasive breast cancer is also present, women are treated as they would be for invasive disease.

I frequently see women whose physicians spoke of and were prepared to treat DCIS as if it were invasive disease. This is unfortunate, because there is a very great difference between an in situ cancer and an invasive one. Although all invasive cancer is thought to arise from preexisting in situ carcinoma, recent studies suggest that only a minority of women who have limited amounts of DCIS ever develop invasive disease, as discussed below. DCIS differs from invasive breast cancer in that it lacks the biological capacity to metastasize. This is an important distinction, because without the capacity to metastasize, DCIS is hardly a cancer as defined by a lay person. To my patients, a cancer (in situ or not) means invasion and potential metastasis. I find it important to take the time to help patients realize the distinction between invasive and in situ disease.

In many institutions, a mastectomy is performed following a diagnosis of DCIS because of two main concerns: a woman might have hidden areas of invasive cancer elsewhere in that breast; or the DCIS may become invasive in time.

First, I will discuss evidence regarding hidden areas of invasion elsewhere in the breast when DCIS is associated with calcifications. The chance of finding invasive cancer appears to be related to the extent of DCIS found. In one study of over ninety women who had a mastectomy for DCIS associated with calcifications, no occult areas of invasive cancer (areas neither seen on the mammogram nor palpated) were present in other parts of the breast when the DCIS was about 45mm or less in size and had been adequately removed (Lagios et al. 1989). As the extent of DCIS increased, so did the likelihood of occult invasion. When the DCIS was 56mm or greater in size, occult invasion was found in 48 percent of the cases. The results of this study suggest that if a woman is diagnosed with DCIS measuring 45mm or less in size, it is unlikely that hidden areas of invasive cancer will also be present in that breast. (Of course, such a woman should have a good physical breast examination and mammograms as well, to make sure there is no evidence of invasive disease elsewhere in the breasts. If invasive breast cancer is present, it should be treated appropriately.)

The second issue to be considered is the chance that invasive breast cancer will develop in the breast following a diagnosis of DCIS. An accurate assessment of this risk is difficult, since mastectomy has been the usual treatment once DCIS is discovered. In one group of twenty-eight women in whom DCIS was overlooked in the initial pathology review, and who therefore received no mastectomy, seven women (25 percent) developed breast cancer over an average follow-up of about seventeen years (Page et al. 1982). Obviously, with only twenty-eight women in the study, the numbers are too small to generalize a risk figure for all women with DCIS. Other studies included only small numbers of women as well. Therefore, at the present time, it appears that once a woman is diagnosed with DCIS, her chance of developing invasive breast cancer in future is somewhat increased, and may depend on the extent and type of disease present, as discussed below.

Size and adequate removal of the DCIS lesion appear to be associated with future risk of invasive disease. In one study, begun in 1971, seventy-nine women whose DCIS was associated with calcifications, and was 25mm in size or smaller, were treated by removing the in situ lesion (with a clear margin around it) and all of the surrounding calcifications. With a median follow-up of sixty-eight months, invasive cancer has occurred in only five women. Five others have developed DCIS. None of the women has developed metastases (Lagios 1990; Lagios et al. 1989).

Pathologists are beginning to classify DCIS by subtype, and are finding preliminary evidence that some subtypes (for example, micropapillary) are less likely to be associated with subsequent invasive or in situ recurrences than are other types (Lagios 1990). Longer follow-up and greater numbers of study subjects are needed to provide definitive risks of recurrence for the different types of DCIS.

At some institutions women with DCIS are treated with radiation therapy. In such cases, future risk of invasive breast cancer appears to be about the same as when complete excision of small lesions is the treatment (Gump 1987; Lagios et al. 1989). To date, studies have small numbers of subjects and have not followed women for long periods of time, so no definitive conclusions about the relative merits of excision or excision plus radiation therapy can yet be reached. Unfortunately, some studies include women with extensive or unknown amounts of DCIS, which increases the probability that invasive cancer was present at the time the DCIS was detected. In most of the studies, it is not known whether the margins were clear—an element that appears to include increased risk of recurrence (Lagios et al. 1989). Further research clearly is needed to establish both estimates of risk and appropriate treatment modalities.

Women in whom DCIS has been diagnosed often assume they have invasive disease. One of my patients in her early fifties, named Karen, was found to have calcifications in her left breast at the time of her first mammogram. Her doctor recommended a biopsy, but she was in the midst of a divorce and was moving, and so did not schedule one for several months. When DCIS was found to be associated with the calcifications in the biopsy specimen, she panicked, and blamed herself terribly for the delay, exclaiming:

> Wouldn't you know it? Just when I have a chance for a new life I go ahead and throw it away by not having a biopsy sooner. Now I'll be holding my breath for the next five years to see if it has spread all over my body.

Karen was convinced that her "breast cancer," as she called it, had already metastasized, and had scheduled appointments with two medical oncologists to begin discussing chemotherapy. When she learned the difference between an in situ and an invasive cancer, she said, "I thought cancer was cancer, and if you didn't get to it within minutes, that was it." I was pleased to be able to tell her that in her case, there was no evidence of invasive disease, and so no evidence of cells that could produce a metastasis.

Once Karen understood the difference between an invasive and in situ breast cancer, she found it easier to think about and discuss treatment options. Her surgeon had told her that mastectomy was usually done when a woman had DCIS, but given the small size of her lesion (about 10mm) and its close association with the calcifications, she could choose instead to be followed carefully by a health care professional. Karen wisely realized that she was hearing a great deal of new information, but was not processing it in a way that would enable her to assess the ramifications of the different choices. I suggested that she bring a friend or relative to the next few meetings, and that we slowly and methodically discuss the various options, giving her time to examine each for a week and see how she felt about it.

At first, Karen felt mastectomy was the only choice that would give her peace of mind. She came to one meeting determined to schedule surgery as soon as possible, so she could "forget all this and get on with my life." Several times she lamented that no one was available to tell her what to do, leading to anxiety and sleepless nights. When family members and I urged her to take her time and postpone surgery until she was sure, she became angry. At one point she and her daughter did not speak for two days.

After several months of soul searching and discussions with friends, family members, and her doctor, Karen decided to be followed closely by a health care professional. In retrospect, she said the anxiety had been worth it. At her last visit, she recalled the anger she initially felt toward me for not encouraging her to have a mastectomy quickly. "Am I glad you hung in there, and urged me to be sure," she said.

Not all women make the decision Karen did. Sara was found to have DCIS when she had a biopsy for a lump in her right breast. No calcifications were present to act as a marker for the presence of DCIS, the DCIS measured well over 40mm, and it extended to the edge of the biopsy specimen. In addition, her breasts were quite lumpy, making them difficult to examine. This was the third biopsy on her right breast, and neither she nor her physician thought the breast would retain a pleasing contour if further tissue were to be removed. She decided, again after a month or so of "agony," as she put it, to have a mastectomy with immediate breast reconstruction.

Linda, a woman in her late fifties, made still a third decision. She had widespread DCIS in her left breast, making it likely that a small area of invasive breast cancer was present. Her breasts were medium-sized, and not difficult to examine. She decided to have radiation treatment to the breast, combined with careful follow-up.

In summary, duct carcinoma in situ (intraductal carcinoma or DCIS) without associated invasive disease will probably be found with increased frequency in the future, as more women have access to mammography, which detects calcifications often associated with this lesion. DCIS differs from invasive breast cancer in that it lacks the biological capacity to metastasize. Limited amounts of DCIS found in association with calcifications have been successfully treated by surgical removal of the DCIS. When DCIS is treated by excision followed by radiation therapy, the likelihood of subsequent development of invasive breast cancer appears to be about the same as when no radiation treatment is used. To date, there are relatively few studies with small numbers of women followed only for limited time periods, so the optimal treatment for DCIS of differing types and extent is not yet known.

Lobular Carcinoma In Situ

Lobular carcinoma in situ (LCIS) is also called lobular neoplasia, a term introduced by Dr. Cushman D. Haagensen in an attempt to clarify the difference between LCIS and invasive lesions. The finding of LCIS is generally fortuitous. That is, a woman has a breast biopsy for a lump or other breast change, and LCIS cells are found during the pathology review. LCIS does not form a lump, nor is it visible on mammograms. It is a diagnosis made by a pathologist following a breast biopsy for other concerns. Therefore, it is likely that this lesion remains undetected in many women who never have a biopsy or who have a part of the breast biopsied that does not contain LCIS.

Dr. Haagensen, who began collecting data on women with LCIS years ago when radical mastectomy was the only standard treatment for invasive breast cancer, did not consider LCIS a true cancer, and so did not recommend a mastectomy for his patients in whom LCIS was found. Instead, he followed over two hundred fifty women with LCIS, some for more than forty years. Thanks to his careful records, as well as his tenacity in keeping track of nearly all study subjects, information is available on the long-term risk of subsequent invasive breast cancer to women with LCIS who do not receive a mastectomy.

In Haagensen's study, risk of invasive disease following a diagnosis of LCIS was found to be about 1 percent a year, when life table analysis was used. In the follow-up which lasted more than thirty-five years, 20 percent developed invasive disease (Haagensen 1986). Haagensen, among others, has found that the risk of invasive disease is not confined to the breast in which LCIS is detected, but is shared equally by both breasts. That is, a woman is just as likely to develop invasive disease in the contralateral breast as in the breast in which the LCIS was found. Instead of developing into invasive cells themselves, LCIS appears to act as a marker for increased risk to both breasts.

Another study which followed fewer than one hundred women with LCIS for a mean of twenty-four years reported that 37 percent subsequently developed invasive breast cancer (Rosen et al. 1978). If those lost to follow-up are assumed to be unaffected, 31 percent developed invasive disease. In this study, the percentage of women affected was used to calculate risk, a method which is less accurate than life table analysis (see Chapter 2). The amount of LCIS was not associated with subsequent risk of invasion (Rosen et al. 1981). That is, women with extensive amounts of LCIS were found to be at no greater risk of developing invasive breast cancer than those with more limited disease. This important discovery suggests that women need not undergo multiple biopsies to remove LCIS.

Women who learn they have LCIS often have uncertainties and concerns about treatment similar to those experienced by women diagnosed with DCIS. Gloria, a woman in her early forties, consulted me following a diagnosis of LCIS. She had been to three different physicians and received three different opinions. None of these physicians suggested she hurry to have treatment, which thoroughly confused her. Gloria had heard her physicians say that she had a precancer. Two physicians suggested further surgery, while one did not. Even the two who thought surgery the best treatment had different approaches. One suggested removal of her left breast, in which LCIS had been found. The other urged her to consider removal of both breasts with immediate reconstruction. When I first saw Gloria, she said:

> I don't really need to discuss risk. Hearing that these cells are precancerous is enough for me. I don't want to fool around with cells like that in my body, waiting for them to turn against me. Whatever it takes, I want to beat this cancer, and I want to start now.

When I asked Gloria what the term precancer meant, she said it was a mild form of cancer that wasn't going to kill her today, but could become a killer at any time. I responded that in my opinion, the term precancer is not useful, since it prejudges a cell. We don't know which, if any, of the cells in an individual's body will become malignant in future, so in this regard, all cells could be called precancerous. I then explained the biological differences between an invasive and an in situ cancer. Gloria had not realized that an in situ cancer lacks the biological capacity to metastasize. "But I seem to have so much of it," she said. "One surgeon said he couldn't get it all out." I then told her of Rosen's study, which found that the amount of LCIS does not appear to influence the subsequent risk of invasive breast cancer. When Gloria considered the risk (about 1 percent a year), she found she could live comfortably with it. "After all," she said, "most of the women with LCIS never get breast cancer, so maybe I won't either. But just in case, I'll be very carefully followed."

Gloria's case demonstrates, as do many others, that words can be more ominous than the cell that is present. For Gloria, the turning point came when she no longer identified herself as a cancer patient. This was difficult for her to do, because one of her friends had advanced breast cancer and was being treated with chemotherapy. This friend, at first not realizing the difference between invasive breast cancer and LCIS, strongly urged Gloria to have both breasts removed as quickly as possible.

Some of the differences between LCIS and DCIS are listed in Table 3-3. Though both are in situ diseases, they have very

Table 3-3. Comparison of In Situ Breast Cancers

Duct Carcinoma In Situ	Lobular Carcinoma In Situ
Can be palpated on breast exam	Cannot be palpated on breast exam
Often detected by calcifications in mammogram	Not detected by mammogram
Risk of invasion depends on extent of disease	Risk of invasion independent of extent of disease
Complete removal advised if no radiation treatment or mastectomy	Complete removal not necessary
Risk to contralateral breast not increased	Risk to contralateral and involved breasts the same

different characteristics, and so may require very different treatment.

In summary, lobular carcinoma in situ (LCIS) or lobular neoplasia is a noninvasive lesion that does not itself appear to metastasize, does not form a lump, and is not seen on mammogram. Its diagnosis is made by a pathologist following a breast biopsy. Women diagnosed with LCIS have a risk of about 1 percent a year of developing invasive breast cancer, with the risk shared equally by both breasts. The amount of LCIS does not appear to influence a woman's risk of subsequent invasive disease.

4

Lifestyle and History

As the public becomes increasingly aware of the links between lifestyle choices, such as diet and smoking, and various diseases, more and more people hope to reduce their risk of disease by making informed choices about these factors. This chapter is largely concerned with lifestyle choices that can be altered—diet, smoking, alcohol consumption. It also discusses reproductive history and stress as they relate to breast cancer risk.

Diet

The results of many studies suggest that diet plays a very significant role in a woman's risk of breast, colon, uterine, and ovarian cancer. Until recent years, there were few scientific studies on diet and breast cancer risk, so much is still unknown in this regard.

Figure 4-1 shows that in Norway, as in the United States, the risk of breast cancer increases with age. In Norway, however, the risk is somewhat lower than in the United States. Generally speaking, the higher the gross national product of a country, the higher the fat consumption—and the higher the risk of breast cancer (Wynder et al. 1986). As also shown,

Figure 4-1. Incidence of Breast Cancer in Women Living in the United States, Norway, and Japan, Periods around 1965

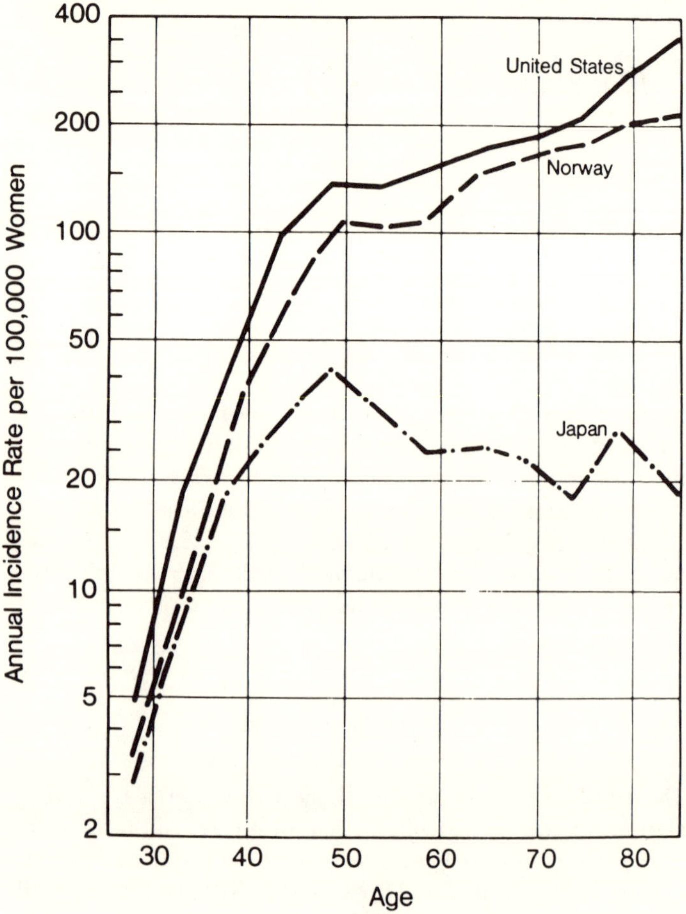

Source: Adapted from Herbert Seidman. 1972. *Cancer of the Breast, Statistical and Epidemiological Data* (New York: American Cancer Society). Reprinted by permission of Herbert Seidman.

the risk of breast cancer in Japan is lower than in the United States and Norway, and does not continue to increase with age. In Japan, 20 percent of the average person's daily diet is composed of fat, compared to 40 percent in the United States. The risk of breast cancer has increased in Japan in recent years, particularly in large cities, where the diet is becoming more Westernized. Among Japanese living in Japan, increased meat consumption is associated with higher risk of breast cancer (Hirayama 1978).

Studies of migrant groups suggest that in large populations environmental factors play a greater role in breast cancer etiology than do genetic factors. For example, Figure 4-2 shows breast cancer rates of Japanese women living in Japan differ from those of Japanese-American women living in Hawaii and the San Francisco Bay area. It is thought that as the Japanese move from Japan to Hawaii, and then to the Bay area, their diet becomes more and more Westernized, with a resulting increase in breast cancer rates. Other environmental factors change as well.

Breast cancer rates also change when other groups migrate, as can be seen in Figure 4-3. At the left, for comparison, is a solid bar showing the breast cancer rate in women born and raised in the United States. For other countries there are two bars: a clear one for the rate in women who remained in the home country, and a shaded one for those who migrated to the United States. In all but one instance (Great Britain), the rate increased when women moved to the United States. In migrants from Great Britain, where the rate was higher than in the United States, a decrease occurred in those who came to the United States.

Another interesting study (see Figure 4-4) found an increase in the breast cancer rate around the world as the average woman's consumption of fat increased (Wynder et al. 1986). Obviously, not all women receive an equal share of fat in any country, so these results are necessarily imprecise. Nevertheless, as Figure 4-4 shows, there is almost a straight-line correlation between the amount of animal fat consumed and the rate of breast cancer.

Figure 4-2. Incidence of Breast Cancer in Japanese Women Living in Japan, Hawaii, and San Francisco Bay Area Compared to Caucasian Women in San Francisco Bay Area, Periods around 1965

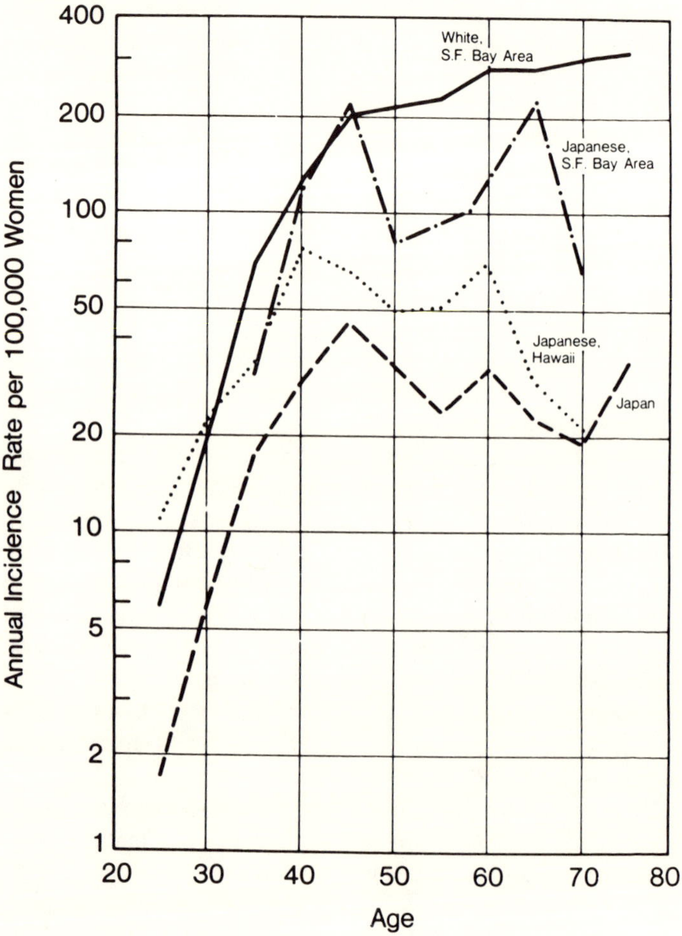

Source: Adapted from P. Buell. 1973. "Changing Incidence of Breast Cancer in Japanese-American Women." *Journal of the National Cancer Institute* 51:1479–1483. Reprinted by permission of the copyright owner, *Journal of the National Cancer Institute.*

Figure 4-3. Changes in Breast Cancer Rates in Immigrants to the United States, 1956–1961

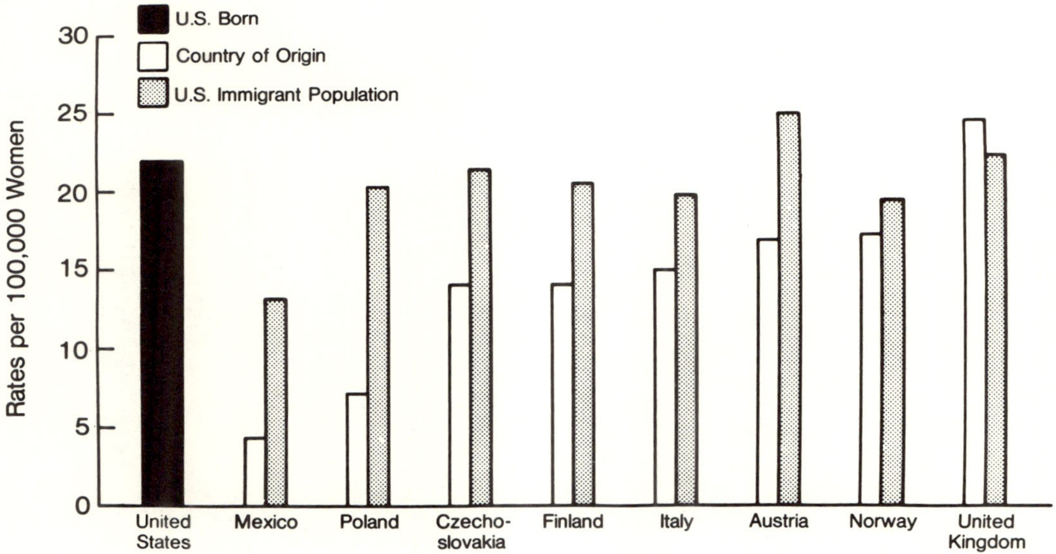

Source: Adapted and reprinted by permission of the publishers from *Cancer in the U.S.: Vital and Health Statistics Monographs* by A. M. Lilienfeld, L. Levin and I. I. Kessler, Cambridge, Mass.: Harvard University Press, Copyright © 1972 by the President and Fellows of Harvard College.

Figure 4-4. Breast Cancer Rates and Per Capita Fat Intake in Women 55 or More Years of Age

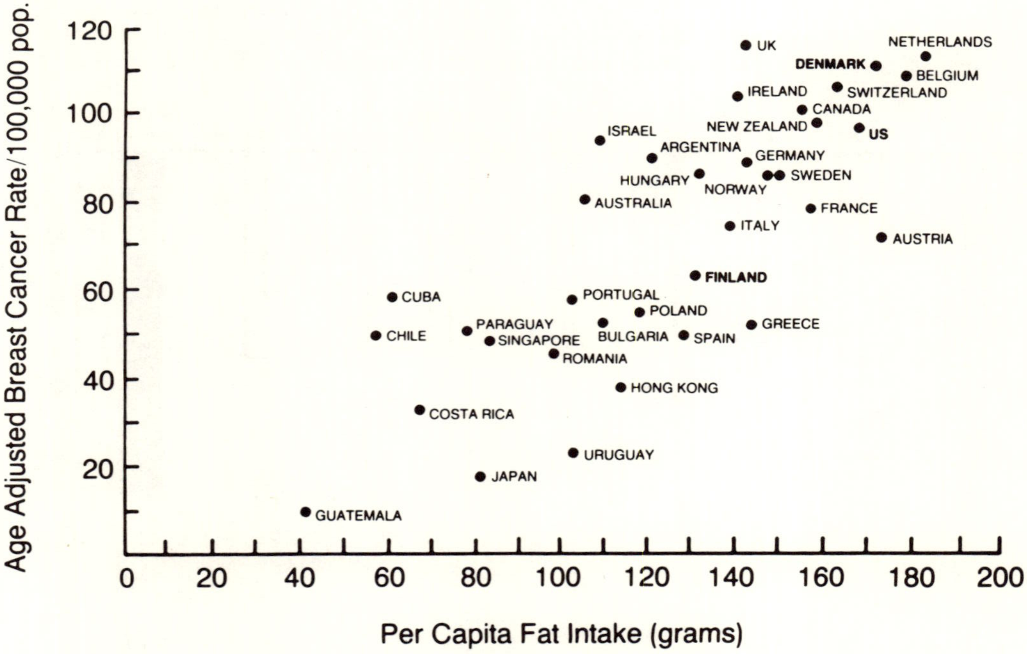

Source: Adapted from E. L. Wynder, et al. 1986. "Diet and Breast Cancer in Causation and Therapy," *Cancer* 58:1804–1813, fig. 4. Reprinted by permission of the copyright owner, *Cancer* and J. B. Lippincott Company.

Finland is an interesting country to note in Figure 4-4, as it has a lower rate of breast cancer than countries with lower or similar rates of fat consumption. Some scientists have suggested that the Finns might receive protection from breast cancer due to the high amounts of fiber in their diets. According to one theory, fiber might hasten the body's elimination of fat, and so reduce its harmful effects. Proponents of another theory note that the Finns consume less fiber than the Danes, yet have a lower rate of both breast and colon cancer. They suggest that the lower Finnish colon cancer rate might be due at least in part to the Finns' higher consumption of fiber containing phytic acid (Graf and Eaton 1985). The consumption of phytic acid might explain the lower rate of breast cancer in the Finns as well. According to the Graf and Eaton theory, phytic acid—which is found in foods such as corn, beans, and whole wheat grains—might protect the body from the cancer-causing effects of oxygen-free radicals which are breakdown products in the digestion of foods, particularly fats.

In one recent and widely reported study of nurses, diet had no apparent effect on risk of breast cancer (Willett et al. 1987a). However, this study's structure was flawed in several important respects, making its conclusions tentative at best. First, subjects were asked to record information about their present and past eating habits. Few individuals can accurately estimate their current food intake, much less that of previous years (Jones et al. 1987), so a lack of association between diet and risk in this study cannot be regarded as definitive. Also, the nurses in this study ranged in age from thirty-four to fifty-nine, and were followed for only four years. Even if they had been able to accurately note their food intake, it is unlikely this short amount of time would be sufficient to show a significant difference in breast cancer rates—particularly if the effects of diet are cumulative and so do not become apparent until later in life.

By comparing the rates of breast cancer in women living in Japan and in the United States (see Figure 4-1), it can be seen that the greatest differences in breast cancer rates appear in older women. This suggests that the effects of diet on breast cancer risk may be greater in older than in younger women. Some studies find a stronger association between fat consumption and breast cancer risk in postmenopausal women than in those who are premenopausal. For example, in one study of over two thousand women, those with a postmenopausal diagnosis of breast cancer were less likely to include vegetables in their diet, particularly vegetables containing beta-carotene, than were women of the same age without such a diagnosis (Graham et al. 1982). In this study, premenopausal women who were and were not diagnosed with breast cancer did not differ significantly in their diets. Individuals were interviewed about their diets retrospectively, so the authors urge caution in interpreting the results.

The age at which an individual begins to eat a low-fat, high-fiber diet may be of great importance. For example, in some studies, adult converts to religious groups having a diet low in fat and high in fiber are found to be at greater risk of breast cancer than are women brought up in the faith, suggesting that the converts changed their diets too late in life to influence risk, or did not change their diets sufficiently (Phillips et al. 1980; Kinlen 1982).

Finally, mice and rats fed a high-fat diet are more likely to develop mammary cancer than are those who are fed less fat (Ip 1980). Studies with animals cannot offer conclusive proof about human beings, of course, but they do lend support to the overall accumulation of evidence. It is interesting to note that fish, olive, and coconut oil did not increase the risk of mammary carcinoma when they comprised less than 40 percent of the calories in the animals' diets (Cohen 1986).

Many patients have heard that diet can affect their risks, but are unsure how seriously to take the information they have heard, or how to effect changes in their own or their family's lives. Individuals may differ greatly in their strategies for improving diet, as two of my patients' experiences demonstrate.

Susan is an attractive, thoughtful woman in her mid forties; she lives with her husband and three daughters, all of whom were accustomed to steak, hamburgers, ice cream, puddings, and snack foods on a regular basis. Susan works outside her home, and so is often exhausted at the end of the day. "I find myself feeding them anything," she said, "just to have them happy and the mealtime over. I want to cook healthy meals, but I don't have the energy at the end of the day." Susan was distressed, because the more she learned about the connection between breast cancer and diet, the more she wanted her daughters to grow up as protected as possible. Also, several of her friends had been diagnosed with breast cancer, so she was increasingly concerned about herself. She realized that a change in diet would not guarantee a reduction in breast cancer risk for her or her daughters, but said, "I know we don't eat well anyway, so it's time for a change. And I want to do something about my breast cancer risk. This is one way for me to feel in control."

Susan and I discussed foods that were high and low in fat (see Table 4-1) and fiber (see Table 4-2), as well as those high in vitamins A, C, and E. Rather than have her march home and declare a new style of eating for her family, which they surely would resist, I suggested that she slowly but surely cut down on the purchase and preparation of foods high in fat, while substituting foods high in fiber. First Susan bought salad materials, and added a salad to the family dinner as a regular component. She says she has added cut vegetables and yogurt dip as an appetizer.

For Susan, as for many busy women, the answer was simplicity and company during meal preparation. She and her family started with salads, then moved on to steamed vegetables. At the same time, she bought fatty meats less often, reduced the portions, and began to "forget" to buy some of the junk food. Without imposing dietary restrictions, she told me that over a six-month period, she had brought about significant healthy changes in her family's diet.

Another patient, Donna, was just as determined and had as little time as Susan, but did not possess the same cooking skills and interests. Donna found herself in an unchanged situation week after week. I suggested she speak with a nutri-

Table 4-1. Fat and Calories from Some Foods

Food	Serving	Calories	Grams of Fat*
American cheese	1 oz	105	9
Cheddar cheese	1 oz	115	9
Cottage cheese	½ cup	115	5
Low-fat cottage cheese	½ cup	100	2
Cream cheese	1 oz	80	5
Parmesan cheese	1 tbsp	25	2
Swiss cheese	1 oz	105	8
Cream	2 tbsp	60	6
Half and half	2 tbsp	40	3
Ice cream	1 cup	270	41
Pot roasted beef	3 oz	255	61
Lean ground beef	3 oz	230	51
Regular ground beef	3 oz	245	71
Roasted chicken, dark	3 oz	175	8
Roasted chicken, light	3 oz	145	4
Egg, hard cooked	1 large	80	6
Baked flounder	3 oz	120	6
Boiled or steamed shrimp	3 oz	100	1
White bread	1 slice	65	1
Pancake, 4 inches	1	60	2
Avocado	½	160	51
Butter, margarine	1 tbsp	100	21
Mayonnaise	1 tbsp	100	21
Oils	1 tbsp	120	41
Peanut butter	1 tbsp	95	8
Salad dressing	1 tbsp	65	6

*If you choose to reduce the fat in your diet to 30 percent of your daily calories, for a 2,000 calorie diet that is about 67 grams of fat. For other foods not listed herein, see Superintendent of Documents, *Nutritive Value of Foods* (Washington, D.C.: U.S. Gov't. Printing Office, n.d.), pamphlet no. HG-72.

Source: U.S. Dept. of Health and Human Services, Public Health Service, "Diet, Nutrition and Cancer Prevention: A Guide To Food Choices" (Washington, D.C.: National Institutes of Health, November 1984), publ. no. 85-2711.

Table 4-2. Fiber Content of Some Foods

Food	Serving	Calories
Rich Sources of Food Fiber		
All Bran*	⅓ cup	70
Bran Buds*	⅓ cup	75
Bran Chex	⅔ cup	90
100% Bran*	½ cup	75
Wheat germ, toasted	¼ cup	110
Blackberries	½ cup	35
Dried prunes	3	60
Moderately Rich Sources of Food Fiber†		
Bran muffins	1	105
Popcorn (air popped)	1 cup	120
Whole wheat bread	1 slice	60
40% Bran Flakes	⅔ cup	90
Oatmeal, cooked	¾ cup	110
Shredded Wheat	⅔ cup	100
Wheaties	1 cup	100
Almonds	10	80
Peanuts	10	105
Artichoke	1 small	45
Asparagus	½ cup	15
Green beans	½ cup	15
Brussels sprouts	½ cup	30
Carrots	½ cup	25
Cauliflower	½ cup	15
Corn	½ cup	70
Green peas	½ cup	55
Potato	1 medium	95

*Six or more grams of fiber per serving.

†1 to 3 grams of fiber per serving.

Source: U.S. Dept. of Health and Human Services, Public Health Service, "Diet, Nutrition and Cancer Prevention: A Guide To Food Choices" (Washington, D.C.: National Institutes of Health, November 1984), publ. no. 85-2711.

tionist, who was able to work with her over a period of time to effect the changes she desired. For Donna, some of the changes involved choosing more wisely at restaurants, and buying low-fat, high-fiber meals at a local take-out restaurant.

Long-lasting eating habits are rarely changed overnight. Instead, someone in the family has to think ahead, plan, and move slowly but surely toward reducing fat and increasing fiber. You may find it useful to remind your patients that the aim is to enjoy the food they eat, as well as to eat in a more healthy manner. Neither they nor their family will long tolerate foods that don't taste good—nor need they do so.

Many of my patients have benefitted from the Diet, Nutrition and Cancer Prevention booklet published by the U.S. Department of Health and Human Services. Some cookbooks also have useful dietary tables. For recipes that are tasty but low in fat and high in fiber, vegetarian cookbooks or those which use the *nouvelle cuisine* approach are often helpful.

Alcohol Consumption

In the last few years, the mass media has widely publicized several studies claiming that even a few drinks of wine a week can significantly increase a woman's risk of breast cancer. These studies suffer from small study group sizes, and generally find very small differences in risk between women who do not drink and those whose drinking practices are moderate. For example, in one study, the drinking habits of 601 women nurses aged thirty-four to fifty-nine who developed breast cancer in a four-year period were compared to those of nearly 89,000 who did not develop breast cancer in the same four years (Willett et al. 1987b). Questionnaires were mailed to women every two years to ask about their alcohol consumption. Very few said they consumed more than three drinks a day.

Table 4-3 shows that women who drank less than 5 grams of wine a day (about half a glass) had a risk of breast can-

Table 4-3. Daily Alcohol Consumption and Breast Cancer Risk*

	Less than Five Grams		Five or More Grams	
Beverage	*Relative Risk*	*Confidence Interval*	*Relative Risk*	*Confidence Interval*
Beer	1.4†	(1.1–1.8)	1.5†	(1.2–2.0)
Wine	1.1	(0.9–1.3)	1.4†	(1.1–1.8)
Liquor	1.1	(0.1–1.3)	1.5†	(1.2–1.9)

*Alcohol content estimated at 13.2 grams for bottle or can of beer, 10.8 grams for glass of wine, and 15.1 grams for a glass of liquor.
†Significant.
Source: W. C. Willett, et al., 1987a. "Dietary Fat and the Risk of Breast Cancer," *New England Journal of Medicine* 316:22–28. Reprinted by permission of the *New England Journal of Medicine.*

cer 1.1 times that of nondrinkers. Those who consumed 5 or more grams of wine a day (more than half a glass) had a risk 1.4 times that of nondrinkers. Note the confidence interval (the numbers in parenthesis next to the relative risk figures). For the relative risk of 1.1, the confidence interval ranges from 0.9 to 1.3. As discussed in Chapter 2, confidence intervals tell you where the true value of the relative risks is likely to be given the information from the study. In this case, for women who drank less than half a glass of wine a day, the confidence interval includes the relative risk of 1.0, which means the observed difference in the number of women with breast cancer in the study and control groups might be due to chance alone.

For those who drank more than half a glass of wine a day, a statistically significant increase in risk was found, but the increase was quite small—a relative risk of 1.4. Remember, also, that the consumption of five or more grams of alcohol a day covers quite a diverse group, ranging from moderate drinkers to alcoholics. This is hardly a precise definition of drinking habits. In Table 4-3 data is presented on those who consume more or less than 5 grams of alcohol a day. The same study also compared risk of breast cancer in women whose alcohol consumption was less than 1.5 grams, 1.5 to 4.9 grams, 5.0 to 14.9 grams, and more than 15.0 grams a day. In this comparison, a significant increase in risk (1.6) was found only when alcohol consumption was greater than 15.0 grams a day. As you can see, by placing the same women in different categories, statistically significant results may appear and vanish.

In another study, current drinkers as a group were not found to be at increased risk of breast cancer compared to nondrinkers (Harvey et al. 1987). An increase in risk was associated instead with drinking habits before age thirty, regardless of current drinking practices. In this study, alcohol consumption might be acting as a marker for another factor that increases risk, since no association with current drinking practices was found. Also, over 80 percent of those who drank at all reported consumption at one or fewer drinks a day, leaving relatively few whose alcohol consumption was high.

A biostatistician colleague, who analyzed a number of these studies, noted that most of the strong associations with risk are found in women whose alcohol consumption is high. At lower levels, great variations are seen. Perhaps even more important, no strong dose effect is seen, again suggesting that alcohol consumption may be a marker for other factors in a person's life, and not the cause of any (or a very small) increase in risk, when consumed in moderate amounts.

Women who drink heavily do appear to be at increased risk of breast cancer (Adelstein and White 1976). However, it is still not clear whether this increase is due to heavy drinking, the poor nutrition that generally accompanies an alcoholic lifestyle, or both. In most studies on alcohol consumption, dietary information is not available.

Many women are confused and disturbed about reports on the effects of moderate alcohol consumption on breast cancer risk, and ask, "What will we next hear is dangerous?" Marcie, who loves to have a glass of wine with her evening meal, was shaken by a newspaper article which stated that even several drinks a week could increase her breast cancer risk by 50 percent. When I showed her that a 50 percent increase in her 1 percent risk over the next ten years would be 1.5 percent in total, or only 0.15 percent a year, she was greatly relieved. I also reminded her that studies to date have by no means shown a clear association between moderate alcohol consumption and breast cancer risk, as discussed above.

At her next visit, however, Marcie asked how many published papers had shown an increase in risk with moderate drinking and how many not. I told her of several which had found no increase in risk (for example, Paganini-Hill and Ross 1983; Webster 1983), and noted that studies which show no association are less likely to be published than are those in which an association is found, particularly if the study group is small. Therefore, as discussed (see Chapter 2's section on publication bias), it is not useful to pile up the numbers of studies on two sides of an issue, and accept the conclusion put forward in the highest stack.

Cigarette Smoking

No clear association between cigarette smoking and breast cancer risk has been established. Many studies show an increased risk of heart disease and upper respiratory cancers in women who smoke, so it is also possible that women develop and die of these diseases first, obscuring any increase in breast cancer risk that might be present. Depending on the study, breast cancer risks to smokers are reported as increased, decreased, or similar to those of nonsmokers (see Brownson et al. 1988). Some investigators find an increase in premenopausal, but not postmenopausal, breast cancer risk in smokers. When an increase in risk is found, it is generally small.

In summary, I think it can be safely said that migrant studies as well as studies on laboratory animals show an association between a diet high in fat and low in fiber with increased breast cancer risk. Still unanswered are questions pertaining to safe levels of fat and fiber consumption, the amount of time that a changed diet must be observed before a significant reduction in risk is found, the ages at which a woman's risk is most susceptible to dietary influences, and the lag time (if any) between a particular dietary change and change in risk. Also unanswered are the ways in which various vitamins, fats, and fibers might interact. Studies on alcohol consumption suggest that heavy drinkers are at increased risk of breast cancer. At moderate levels the risks are either not increased or increased only slightly. No clear association has been found between cigarette smoking and breast cancer risk.

Reproductive History

Many women have heard that their risk of breast cancer is increased if they are nulliparous (never gave birth) or gave birth to their first child at an older age. Some express concern about their age at menarche or menopause, having heard that these also affect a woman's breast cancer risk. Some studies do find that reproductive history factors are associated with differences in breast cancer risk, but not to the extent that most women believe.

Parity

Many older studies reported that increased parity or increased number of children born was associated with decreased breast cancer risk. More recent studies have shown it is not the number of children, but the age at which a first child is born, that is of importance. Women with a greater number of children are more likely to have their first child at an earlier age, and appear to be at lower risk because they start childbearing earlier (MacMahon et al. 1970). Most large studies in the United States and around the world find an association between breast cancer risk and a woman's age at the time of her first live birth (stillbirths and miscarriages do not appear to influence the risk of developing breast cancer). In some studies, women who give birth to their first child after thirty years of age are at higher risk than those who are nulliparous (Brinton et al. 1982; MacMahon et al. 1970).

In speaking to women about risk due to reproductive history, I like to use the results of the Brinton et al. study (1982) because it is based on large numbers of women from around the country and analyzes risk separately for women who did and did not have a mother or sister with breast cancer. Although distinctions between different types of family history were not made, and paternal family history was not considered, this was one of the first studies on reproductive history to include family history in a meaningful manner. (See Chapter 6 for a discussion of the importance of different types of family history.)

Analysis of Dr. Brinton's data shows that women who have no mother or sister with breast cancer, and who first bear children at age thirty and over, have a risk twice that of women who first bear children between the ages of twenty and twenty-four. The risk to nulliparous women is somewhat less—1.3. A more recent report constructed what the authors called a risk model to estimate risk in the same population originally studied by Dr. Brinton (Gail et al. 1989). When compared to children who had their first child before age twenty, those who first gave birth from twenty to twenty-four had a relative risk of 1.2, while those who were twenty-five to twenty-nine or nulliparous (the researchers' combined category) had a relative risk of 1.5. Those thirty and older had a relative risk of 1.9.

Present day studies of risk to age sixty or seventy are, of course, based on women who became pregnant some years ago, when women tended to marry and give birth at younger ages than do some groups of women today. It has not yet been shown that the increase in risk with older age at first birth applies to the many women today who choose to wait to have their first child or who choose to be nulliparous. In the past, the comparatively few women who waited to have a first child may have had other characteristics which also predisposed them to breast cancer.

One recent study analyzed the risk of breast cancer in over eight hundred women who were treated for infertility (Cowan et al. 1981). Progesterone-deficient women were five times as likely to be diagnosed with premenopausal breast cancer than were women who had no hormonal problems. No significant difference in risk of postmenopausal breast cancer was found between the two groups. A recent Israeli study failed to find a significant increase in risk of breast cancer in either infertile women considered as a group, or women with a hormonal deficiency (Ron et al. 1987). The number of subjects in both these studies is small (less than fifty in any subgroup), so their results cannot be considered conclusive. I mention them here, since they suggest that more precise studies, which take into account the reason for older age at birth of a first child or nulliparity, may show that not all subgroups are at increased risk or may be at less risk than previous studies have suggested.

Age at Menarche

In many studies, women in whom menarche started before age twelve are found to be at higher risk of breast cancer than those who started at later ages (Haagensen et al. 1981; Henderson et al. 1974; Yuasa and MacMahon 1970), but this is not found by others (Wynder et al. 1978; Adami et al. 1978). In one study, an association between early menopause and increased risk of premenopausal, but not postmenopausal, disease was found (Stavraky and Emmons 1974). The accuracy of such studies is obviously only as precise as a woman's memory. Many, for example, may remember that they were "about twelve" at the time of menarche, without remembering their exact age. For others, the memory is more clear, either because it is associated with a particular event, or because they were considerably older or younger than their peers.

Brinton et al. (1982) found relative risk of breast cancer decreased as age at menarche increased. However, differences in risk between those under age twelve at menarche and those age fourteen and older were found to be very little—an estimated 1 percent to age seventy. No significant differences were found between cases and controls when the age groups less than twelve and fourteen and older were calculated separately, although a significant trend over time was present. A more recent report made use of data from this study, and so obtained similar results (Gail et al. 1989). When compared to women with menarche at age fourteen, those with menarche at twelve to thirteen and less than twelve were found to have relative risks of 1.1 and 1.2 respectively.

As Haagensen (1981) notes, the results of these studies are difficult to interpret, since the average age at menarche has decreased at a rate of about four months every ten years. In 1981, the average age at menarche in the United States was about 12.8 years. Some of this decrease in age could be due to changes in diet, which also influence risk of breast cancer (see discussion earlier in this chapter). In this way, one risk factor may be linked with another, making it difficult to disentangle the effect of each.

Age at Menopause

Women who start menopause after age fifty-five are found to be at somewhat increased risk of breast cancer in some studies (e.g., Haagensen 1981; Trichopoulos et al. 1972), but by no means in all (Salber et al. 1969; Bulbrook 1976). Brinton et al. (1979) found a significant association between breast cancer risk and natural menopause only in those whose menopause occurred at age fifty-five or older. In this group the risk was 2.2 times that of women whose natural menopause occurred at ages forty-five to forty-nine. In women who had a surgical menopause, only those whose menopause occurred at ages forty-five to forty-nine were found to have a significant increase in risk—1.7 compared to women the same age who had a natural menopause. These results differ from Haagensen (1981), who found women who had an oophorectomy (removal of ovaries) to be at decreased risk of breast cancer, with the lowest risk in those who had removal at younger ages. The differences in the two studies' findings may be due to relatively small differences in risk, small sample sizes, differences in women who had surgical menopause over time, as well as differences in study design. In Brinton's study, control groups were composed of women who chose to take part in a national screening program, and so differed from women in the general population who comprised the control groups in Haagensen's and most other studies investigating this issue.

Family History and Reproductive Factors

For some years, scientists speculated about the effects of combined risk factors on a woman's risk of breast cancer. Some proposed addition of risks, while others felt multiplication was warranted. Dr. Brinton's studies suggest that for family history and reproductive history, the combined effects are additive, at most. Compared to women who have no mother or sister with breast cancer, and who have their first child between the ages of twenty and twenty-four, those with an affected relative have a two- to threefold increase in risk if they have their first child before age thirty or are nulliparous. Those whose first child was born when they were thirty or older had a relative risk of 3.8, but there were relatively few women in this category, so these results are far from definitive. These figures are obviously not accurate for all women with a family history of breast cancer, since paternal history was not included, nor was age at diagnosis or the type of family history taken into account (see Chapter 6).

A recent study that constructed a model of risk attempted to make use of family history, but had access only to information on maternal history (Gail et al. 1989). Relative risks for this group, compared to those with no mother or sister with breast cancer, were 2.6 for those who bore a first child before age twenty, 2.7 for first birth at age twenty to twenty-four, and 2.8 for age twenty-five and older or nulliparous. These relative risks are within the range found in studies on family history alone (see Chapter 6). Calculations were made for women with two or more affected relatives, but with fewer than fifty cases and twenty-five controls in any age group, the results are not clinically useful.

Another recent study, which analyzed the effects of type of family history (see Chapter 6 for a description of these types) and reproductive history, found that among women whose sisters had unilateral breast cancer, those who started menarche at an earlier age were at a greater risk of breast cancer than those who started at an older age (Anderson and Badzioch 1989). Age at birth of first child did not appear to significantly influence breast cancer risk. No meaningful information was available on nulliparous women. The number of sisters at risk in each of the groups studied was relatively small, so these results are suggestive and not definitive.

Breast-feeding

Studies on breast-feeding generally suffer methodologically by either relying on women's memories about the length of time they breast-fed, or simply asking women whether or not they breast-fed, disregarding the amount of time they did so. Some studies find that breast cancer risk is somewhat decreased in women who breast-fed, while others find no such difference (for example, Wynder et al. 1978). In a recent study that did ask about the length of time breast-feeding occurred, those who had ever breast-fed were at significantly less risk of premenopausal, but not postmenopausal, breast cancer (McTiernan and Thomas 1986). When length of time was considered, duration of four or more months was associated with a significant decrease in risk. The numbers of women studied are small, and the control groups were drawn from the general population, so these results are preliminary.

In summary, differences in childbearing history and age at menarche and menopause are associated with differences in breast cancer risk in many but not all studies. In most instances, when differences are found, the effects of these factors on an individual woman's risk appear to be rather low—that is, less than twofold. In most studies, parous women are at less risk than those who are nulliparous, but reasons for nulliparity have not been considered. Early age at birth of a first child appears to reduce risk, but these results are based on populations whose reproductive decisions and options differed from those of many modern women. Reproductive decisions may be a marker for different lifestyles, each with different factors influencing risk. In short, these studies may have limited applicability to women today.

At least one study of progesterone-deficient women suggests this group might be at increased risk of breast cancer, but this finding awaits further confirmation. A decrease in risk of premenopausal breast cancer was found in women who breast-fed four or more months, but additional studies are needed in this area as well.

Stress and Personality

When I first began to investigate the possible effects of stress and personality on a woman's breast cancer risk, I thought I would find a great deal of scientific evidence showing a strong connection. It seemed plausible that stress and personality factors would reduce the efficiency of a person's immune system, and so help to bring about breast cancer. Studies showing that the mind affects the body and the body influences the workings of the mind seemed further to suggest a causal relationship between emotions, personality, and the etiology of breast cancer.

I soon learned how difficult it is to devise scientific studies in this area, since clear, scientific measurements of different stress and personality types are not yet available. Moreover, there are as yet no ways to measure the effects of the same stress on different people, or even the effects of the same stress on the same person at different times. Obviously, to some people, stress is like seasoning in food—it makes life interesting. To others, the same stress may be experienced as an overseasoned dish that reduces enjoyment of the taste. This is an important distinction, since the level of stress appears to be less important than the way in which an individual deals with it (Fox 1983; Sklar and Anisman 1981).

Methodological problems are glaringly evident in many studies that attempt to determine the relationship between stress, personality, and cancer. In most, the numbers studied are too small to produce meaningful results. As Fox (1983) notes, even when a large group is studied, cancers of different types are often included (for example, Dattore et al. 1980; Thomas et al. 1979). The etiology of different cancers appears to be influenced by very different genetic and environmental factors, so it is unlikely that studies combining these different diseases will be able to provide useful information about the effects of stress and personality.

Many of my patients express concern that stress will bring about breast cancer, fearing that their very concern is increasing risk. This fear, of course, often intensifies their stress level. I find patients and health professionals tend to be less informed about studies that find no association between stress and personality than about those that do. For example, one study, which used a life-events questionnaire covering the preceding three years, found that women diagnosed with breast cancer or benign breast disease experienced fewer stressful events than the control group did (Priestman et al. 1985). In another instance, a prospective study that used the Minnesota Multiphasic Personality Inventory (MMPI) and included over 8,900 women followed from 1969 to 1988 found no association between depression and a breast cancer diagnosis (Hahn and Petitti 1988). All women in this study belonged to a prepaid health plan, so members of the control group were just as likely to have breast cancer detected as were study subjects. The size and methodology of this study are also impressive.

Patients are sometimes incredulous when they first hear

there is no clear scientific evidence that stress or personality type cause cancer. Many look back to times in their own or others' lives that appear to be causative. As one said:

> If the stress at my job didn't do it, what did? I have to know what caused my cancer, so I know what to change to keep it from coming back.

In such cases, I find patients are helped by learning about the difference between an etiologic agent and one that could be a promoter after the event.

Fox (1983) has written a most thoughtful review of the methodological problems associated with studies in this area, and has carefully weighed what can now be said about the role of psychological factors and stress in cancer etiology and prognosis. He concludes that if personality and stress do affect risk of developing cancer, their influence is small. Susan Sontag's (1979) insights and historical comparisons regarding the ways in which our society has viewed tuberculosis and cancer are quite useful to patients. For example, she notes:

> Theories that diseases are caused by mental states and can be cured by willpower are always an index of how much is not understood about the physical terrain of a disease. [Sontag, 1979, 54]

At the present time, overall, there is no clear-cut scientific evidence that a particular personality type or a stressed life predisposes an individual woman to develop breast cancer. Instead, it appears that if stress and personality type are associated with an increased risk of breast cancer, the personality types and stresses have not yet been adequately defined.

5

Exogenous Hormones

The long-term effects of exogenous hormone use are of great concern to women and health professionals. In this chapter, results of studies on breast cancer risk and oral contraceptives, hormone replacement therapy at menopause, and DES are discussed.

Oral Contraceptives

American women began to use hormones for birth control in 1960, with an estimated 19 percent of those aged fifteen to forty-five taking some type of hormone for birth control by 1975 (Paul et al. 1986). Since the 1960s, twenty different types of oral contraceptives have been used, with the dose steadily declining over time. These temporal changes make it difficult to compare the results of different studies, particularly those in which dose and duration of use are not specified. The results of early studies also were limited by their small samples and lack of follow-up.

More recent studies, which have been able to include larger numbers of long-term users and which generally specify the amount and type of oral contraceptive, generally find no increased risk of breast cancer to previous or current users.

Even women who took oral contraceptives for long periods of time, who started before age twenty, or who had other risk factors such as a family history of breast cancer, are not found to be at increased risk of breast cancer in many well-designed studies.

In preparing this chapter, which reviews some of the larger and better known studies of breast cancer risk in oral contraceptive users, I was again impressed by the lack of data showing a significant association between oral contraceptive use and breast cancer risk. The terms increase and no increase in risk used in describing study results refer to those in which a significant difference was found. (See Chapter 2 for a discussion of significance.)

A nationwide endeavour conducted by the Centers for Disease Control and the National Institute of Child Health and Human Development compared oral contraceptive use among nearly five thousand women diagnosed with breast cancer and a similar number without such a diagnosis (Sattin et al. 1986). In this study, type of oral contraceptive use was carefully noted, as was age at first use, duration of use, length of time since last use, and other factors such as family history. In short, this was a most comprehensive study. No increase in breast cancer risk was found between women who took oral contraceptives and those who did not, regardless of type. Neither duration of use nor length of time since last use was associated with increased risk. Those who started using oral contraceptives before age twenty or before a first pregnancy were not found to be at increased risk of breast cancer. Finally, those who belonged to subgroups already at increased risk of breast cancer (for example, family history of breast cancer or benign breast disease), did not experience further increases in risk due to oral contraceptive use.

Another study, which included over two thousand women diagnosed with breast cancer before age forty-five and two thousand without such a diagnosis, found no association between oral contraceptive use and breast cancer risk (Stadel et al. 1985). Even those whose use began before age twenty, or before a first pregnancy, and whose duration of use was four or more years were not at increased risk of breast cancer. The number of women included in most of the subgroups was large, with the exception of those whose use started before age twenty-five.

A New Zealand study (Paul 1986) is of interest, because it made use of all women aged twenty-five to fifty-four who were diagnosed with breast cancer in that country between July 1983 and June 1985. In New Zealand, an estimated 35 percent of the women aged fifteen to forty-five had taken oral contraceptives, so there was a large group on which data was available. In this study, users were diagnosed with breast cancer at the same age as nonusers, suggesting that oral contraceptives did not significantly speed the growth of an already existing cancer. As a group, users were not at increased risk of breast cancer compared to nonusers. No increase in risk was found in women whose use started before age twenty or before a first pregnancy. Use for ten or more years also was not associated with an increased breast cancer risk. The relative risk to users aged twenty-five to thirty-four was found to be 2.2, and was widely reported as evidence that birth control pills increase risk of breast cancer to women in this age group. However, this finding was based on only forty cases and one hundred eighty-two controls, and the difference was *not* significant.

A different type of study compared prognosis in women with breast cancer who had and had not taken oral contraceptives (Rosner and Lane 1986). Prognosis was not found to be significantly influenced by previous or recent use, suggesting that oral contraceptive use did not activate or significantly promote growth of existing breast cancer cells.

Several studies in the last year have again raised concerns about oral contraceptive use, particularly in younger women. One British study investigated risk of breast cancer to women before age thirty-six (Chilvers et al. 1989). As the authors note, but others tend to overlook, this is a very limited group, and contains limited numbers. In this study, a trend of significantly increased risk was found with increasing duration of use. As a group, parous and nulliparous women also showed a significant trend in increased risk with increased use. For parous women, trend in increased risk was found if use started either before or after a first pregnancy. However, when both duration of use and age at start of use were taken into account, no significant increase in risk was found. This finding is puzzling, since one would also expect a significant increase in risk here if oral contraceptive use were actually increasing breast cancer risk. Further, confidence intervals are not generally given for subgroups within this study, leaving one to wonder about their significance levels. The authors state that oral contraceptive users were more likely to be seen for a medical examination than nonusers, and thus more likely to be carefully screened and diagnosed. At least some of the difference between the study and control groups is likely to be due to this bias.

Another recent British study received much publicity, and caused great concern, when it reported a 3.3 times increase in breast cancer risk to oral contraceptive users aged thirty to thirty-four (Kay and Hannaford 1988). However, those aged twenty-five to twenty-nine were not at significantly increased risk, nor was an increase in risk found when all women younger than age thirty-five were considered. Given these disparate findings, it is important to remember that as discussed in Chapter 2, a significant difference is obtained 5 percent of the time when two groups differ by chance alone. In this instance, the increased risk in the thirty to thirty-four-year-old group may well be due to chance. Even if this difference is not due to chance, and other studies that report no increase in risk to women in this age group are in error, the actual risk to this group, as reported in the paper itself, is one in seven thousand women a year. Once again, a significant risk turns out to be quite a low numerical risk of developing breast cancer.

In summary, most recent, well-constructed studies find no significant association between the use of oral contraceptives and breast cancer risk. Oral contraceptive users who have benign breast disease or a family history of breast cancer do not appear to further increase their risk of developing breast cancer. Women who use oral contraceptives do not develop breast cancer at younger ages than nonusers, nor does oral contraceptive use appear to influence a woman's prognosis if she should develop breast cancer.

Some studies have found an increased risk to subgroups of users. However, the subgroups are generally small and are not consistent from study to study, suggesting that much or all of the increase found is due to methodological problems or chance. There might be subgroups at somewhat increased risk, but these have not yet been identified. In one recent study, a 3.3 times relative risk to women aged twenty-five to twenty-nine was found to be one in seven thousand a year in numerical terms.

Questions remain about oral contraceptive use of twenty or more years, as well as risk to women whose use stopped over twenty years ago, since sufficient data on women in these categories are not yet available for study. More information is also needed on the effects of oral contraceptives in very young women (Shapiro 1986). Information about these groups will be available in time, as larger numbers accumulate. At present, it appears that if there is an increase in breast cancer risk to women who use oral contraceptives, it is quite small.

Replacement Hormones

Since 1942, estrogens have been prescribed in the United States as replacement hormones following natural or surgically induced menopause. However, it was not until the 1960s that large numbers of American women began using replacement estrogens. By 1983 an estimated 2.3 million women were using some type of replacement hormone (Wingo et al. 1987).

Among those using replacement estrogens alone (ERT), the risk of developing, but not dying of, endometrial carcinoma was found to be increased (Astedt 1987). The death rate apparently was not increased because women using replacement hormones were followed by a physician, leading to early detection of carcinomas that did develop. Also, the type of endometrial (uterine) cancer that occurred was slow growing and did not tend to metastasize. To reduce the risk of endometrial cancer, physicians have increasingly prescribed a replacement regimen containing both an estrogen and a progestin. A number of recent studies finds no increase in risk of endometrial carcinoma in women taking an estrogen and progesterone combination at menopause. Some even report a reduction in risk (Astedt 1987).

The use of both estrogen and progesterone is relatively recent, so most studies investigating the risk of breast cancer in women taking replacement hormones have dealt primarily with estrogens only, and in higher doses than would be prescribed today. Therefore, recent studies that report on the effects of fifteen or twenty years of hormone use may give different results than studies published twenty years from now. Meanwhile, as more women take replacement hormones, the number of subjects available for study continues to increase.

One study of over eighteen hundred women who took replacement estrogens found no significant difference in breast cancer risk between users and nonusers (Hoover et al. 1976). During the average follow-up of twelve years, forty-nine of these women developed breast cancer. No significant increase in risk was found with use up to fourteen years. Women who used replacement hormones for fifteen or more years had a twofold increase in risk of breast cancer, which was significant.

In this study, subjects were from higher socioeconomic groups than those in the control group, who were drawn from the general population. Since women from higher socioeconomic groups have an increased risk of breast cancer whether they take replacement hormones or not, the increase in risk to those using replacement hormones for more than fifteen years could be due to this bias. Another bias, of course, arises from the use of the general population as controls, since individuals in this group generally have less access to physicians than those in the study group, and so are less likely to have an existing breast cancer diagnosed.

A study without these biases was conducted by Dr. Louise Brinton and colleagues who studied risk of breast cancer to over 1,900 users of replacement hormones and 2,258 nonusers (Brinton et al. 1986). All of these women took part in a national screening program in which they received mammograms and physician examinations on a regular basis. Therefore, detection of breast cancer in both groups was likely to be similar. In this prospective study, women who took replacement hormones were not found to be at increased risk of developing breast cancer when compared to those who did not. No significant increase in risk was found with use up to twenty years, with risk to users and nonusers compared in four-year increments. A trend test (that is, one testing for significance over time) showed a small but significant increase, estimated to be about 2 percent to women aged sixty-five to seventy-nine who used estrogen for fifteen or more years. No significant increase in risk was found among those whose known dose was increased, even to levels four times greater than that generally prescribed today.

Women with a family history of breast cancer were not at further increased risk if they took replacement hormones, nor were nulliparous women, nor those who had a breast biopsy. Women whose use started after a first breast biopsy did have a significant increase in risk with ten or more years of use, but one of the comparison groups consisted of fewer than twenty women, and as noted in Chapter 3, women with benign breast disease are a heterogenous group, so the clinical relevance of this finding is not clear.

The stage of a woman's breast cancer at time of diagnosis was not significantly associated with use, suggesting that replacement hormones did not cause existing cancers to grow more rapidly in users than in nonusers. In situ cancers and invasive cancers smaller than 1 cm were more likely to be found among long-term users than were larger invasive cancers. Again, the number of women in each group is small, so the clinical importance of these findings is difficult to assess at present.

One recent British study of over forty-five hundred women included those who received either estrogen only or a com-

Table 5-1. Replacement Estrogen Use and Risk of Developing Cancer

Site	Relative Risk	Confidence Interval
Endometrium (uterus)	2.8*	(1.5–5.0)
Breast	1.6*	(1.2–2.1)
Ovary	0.9	(0.3–1.9)
Cervix	0.5	(0.1–1.7)

*Significant.
Source: Kathryn Hunt, et al., 1987. "Long-term Surveillance of Mortality and Cancer Incidence in Women Receiving Hormone Replacement Therapy," *British Journal of Obstetrics and Gynecology* 94:620–635. Reprinted by permission of the copyright owner, *British Journal of Obstetrics and Gynecology*.

bination of both estrogen and progestin for a mean of sixty-seven months (Hunt et al. 1987). Those who took both hormones received far less progestin than would be given today, thereby lessening the effectiveness of this regimen, and probably accounting for a higher incidence of uterine cancer than would be found if a modern regimen were used. As shown in Table 5-1, women taking replacement hormones had a significantly higher risk of breast and endometrial cancers than those in the general population to whom they were compared. (The risks of cervical and ovarian cancers were not significantly reduced—that is, differences between the groups that did and did not take replacement hormones were not greater than those expected by chance alone. For a discussion of significance, see Chapter 2.) Women in this study who took replacement hormones were from higher socioeconomic groups than the control population, which may account for the increased rates in these groups.

Table 5-2 reports mortality rates found in the same groups just discussed. Note the significant reduction in death rate due to breast cancer among those who took replacement hormones. It is not likely that replacement hormones are

Table 5-2. Replacement Estrogen Use and Risk of Death Due to Cancer and Other Diseases

Cause of Death	Relative Risk	Confidence Interval
Endometrial cancer	—	—
Breast cancer	0.5*	(0.28–0.96)
Ovarian cancer	1.1	(0.5–2.2)
Cervical cancer	0.5	(0.1–1.9)
Other cancers	0.7	(0.5–1.0)
Heart disease	0.5*	(0.3–0.7)
All circulatory diseases	0.5*	(0.4–0.7)

*Significant.
Source: Kathryn Hunt, et al., 1987. "Long-term Surveillance of Mortality and Cancer Incidence in Women Receiving Hormone Replacement Therapy," *British Journal of Obstetrics and Gynecology* 94:620–635. Reprinted by permission of the copyright owner, *British Journal of Obstetrics and Gynecology*.

responsible for this decrease. Instead, those who took hormones were probably followed more carefully by a physician or nurse, and so were less likely to have an advanced breast cancer at the time of diagnosis. As shown in Table 5-2, heart disease and deaths due to circulatory diseases were also significantly decreased in women taking replacement hormones. As discussed below, other studies also find a reduction in deaths due to these diseases in postmenopausal women who take replacement hormones.

Another recent study has found that among women diagnosed with breast cancer at age fifty or older, those who were taking replacement estrogens prior to their diagnosis had a significantly improved survival compared to nonusers (Bergkvist et al. 1989). The authors of this study suggest that breast cancers might be found at an earlier stage in women taking replacement estrogens due to closer medical supervision.

In a study with a hospital-based control group, estrogen replacement therapy use was compared in over sixteen hundred women with breast cancer and a similar number admitted to the hospital without such a diagnosis (Kaufman et al. 1984). As a group, those who had taken estrogen replacement therapy were not at increased risk of breast cancer. No increase in risk was found in subgroups thought to be susceptible to hormones (for example, those with a family history of breast cancer or with benign breast disease).

This study also investigated the timing of replacement hormone use in regard to the subsequent diagnosis of breast cancer. No significant difference in use of hormones in the eighteen months prior to hospital admission or use before this time was found between the study and control group. Similarly, no difference was found in women whose use started within ten years of hospital admission, had stopped prior to ten years before admission, or whose use spanned ten or more years before admission. These results suggest that replacement hormones do not cause sudden growth in an existing breast cancer cell. The question of estrogen's ability to stimulate an already existing tumor cell deserves more investigation, using nonhospital-based control groups, since different hospitals attract different types of patients, which could lead to unidentified differences between the study and control groups. Even when members of a control group are chosen from several different hospitals, one cannot be sure they represent the general population. For these reasons, hospital control groups are less reliable than those chosen from the population at large (see Feinstein 1988).

Another study of over thirteen hundred women with breast cancer and sixteen hundred without found no significant increase in risk of breast cancer with replacement hormone use of twenty or more years (Wingo et al. 1987). However, after twenty years there were fewer than thirty women in the study and control groups. Women with a family history of breast cancer, nulliparous women, and those with benign breast disease were not found to be at significantly increased risk if they took replacement hormones.

A Swedish study created quite a stir in 1989 when it reported an increase in breast cancer risk to women who took replacement hormones compared to women in the general population (Bergkvist et al. 1989). Many thought thousands of women were studied. Actually, from a group of twenty-three thousand women who took replacement hormones and who were followed for a mean of 5.7 years, 638 responded to a questionnaire. Of these, 196 women with invasive and 11 with in situ breast cancer formed the study group, with from 1 to 5 control women chosen who had not used replacement hormones or who had used them for 6 months or less. The size of this study was therefore adequate, but less than many others. As a group, women taking replacement hormones had a risk not significantly different from those who did not take such hormones. However, among women whose use was 109 months or longer, users had a relative risk of 2.3, which was significant.

The authors also analyzed risk by type of hormone used—estradiol compounds, conjugated estrogens, and other estrogens. A significant increase in risk was found only for the group who took estradiols for 73 to 109 months, but not for other periods of time. No increase in risk was found in those who took conjugated estrogens, the type most often prescribed in the United States. The findings in this Swedish study may, therefore, not be applicable to most women in the United States who take replacement hormones.

Although much has been written about this study, few seem to have commented on the obvious—fewer than two hundred women with invasive disease comprised the study group, and two of the three hormone preparations studied differed from those generally prescribed in the United States. Also, no trend for increased risk was found over time for two of the three hormone preparations, nor was a significant difference present when different time intervals were analyzed separately for either conjugated or other estrogens. Finally, in this study, the control group consisted of women in the general population, in whom breast cancer can be expected to be diagnosed at a lower frequency than in the study population. In reviewing this study, I am impressed with the number of nonsignificant results that were reported, given the large number of comparisons made. The larger the number of comparisons made, the greater the likelihood of obtaining significant associations that are due to chance alone, as discussed in Chapter 2.

A number of studies have now shown that replacement hormones reduce the risk of osteoporosis (for example, Weiss et al. 1980; Hutchinson et al. 1979; Kreiger et al. 1982). In most studies the risks of coronary disease are also reduced in hormone replacement users (for example, Gordon 1978; Henderson et al. 1988; Stampfer et al. 1985; Bush et al. 1983), but this result has not been found by all investigators, particularly in case-control studies (for example, Wilson et al. 1985), which suffer from the biases discussed in Chapter 2. This probable reduction in risk is important, since coronary heart diseases cause more deaths than all cancers combined (Bayliss et al. 1987). In 1983, for example, five hundred thousand women died from cardiovascular diseases (Bush et al. 1983) compared to an estimated thirty-seven thousand who died of breast cancer (Silverberg and Lubera 1983). Hormone replacement therapy may also offer protection from mortality due to stroke. In a study of over eight thousand women in a retirement community, those who took replacement estrogens were half as likely to die of stroke (Paganini-Hill et al. 1988). The difference was significant.

I see many women who have decided not to take replacement hormones because they fear these hormones will cause them to develop breast cancer. They are unaware of the large, carefully constructed studies whose findings suggest that women in the United States who take replacement hormones in the combinations typically prescribed in this country have no increased risk or very little increased risk of developing this disease even with twenty years of use. At the same time, many studies have shown that postmenopausal women who do not take replacement hormones are at increased risk of heart disease and osteoporosis, diseases that are serious threats to older women's health and lives.

Some who initially reject hormone replacement therapy due to fear of breast cancer reconsider their decision when the effects of hormone reduction seem overwhelming, and when they learn more about the studies discussed above. Phyllis is a woman in her early seventies whose sister was diagnosed with breast cancer in her late fifties. Phyllis said she suffered such vaginal dryness that at times she could hardly walk. Various creams and lubricants prescribed by her doctor were of little use. She was referred to me by a new doctor she began seeing when her previous physician moved to another city.

At first Phyllis did not want to discuss the risks and benefits of replacement therapy, stating, "I don't want to hear anything that will frighten me." She was very relieved to learn of the studies discussed above that generally find little or no increase in risk of breast cancer with years of use, even in women who have a family history of breast cancer. As Phyllis put it, "I thought replacement hormones were guaranteed to give me breast cancer, especially with my sister having it. But I don't mind taking some risk to improve the quality of my life." Phyllis scheduled an appointment with her doctor the day after her final visit with me. Several months later she called to say that since starting hormone replacement therapy, she felt like a new woman and was once again able to take hikes with her family.

When Sally, a woman in her early fifties, started menopause, hot flashes were causing her considerable embarrassment and discomfort at work. In addition, she found that for the first time in her life, little problems would cause her to weep. Since she is a woman who prides herself on order and control, these were difficult symptoms to endure. Sally did not wish to take hormone replacement therapy for several reasons: she had heard it increased the risk of breast cancer, and she felt she wanted to live "naturally" and "in harmony with nature." She felt that if nature had intended her to take hormones, they would have been provided. After we talked it over, Sally realized that what nature provides can be insufficient, as in the need for eyeglasses with age.

In summary, studies with large control and study groups have generally found that women who take estrogen replacement therapy are at little or no increased risk of breast cancer with up to twenty years of use. The risk might be slightly increased after this time, but sufficient numbers are not yet available to be conclusive. Women with benign breast disease or a family history of breast cancer do not appear to further increase their risk of breast cancer by taking replacement hormones. As a group, these studies suggest that hormone replacement therapy either does not increase risk of breast cancer, does so to a very small extent, or may influence the risk to particular subgroups that have not yet been identified. Further, the health benefits from replacement therapy may outweigh the risks.

DES (Diethylstilbestrol)

DES, or diethylstilbestrol, is a synthetic estrogen that was prescribed, primarily between 1940 and 1970, to prevent miscarriage. Studies in 1953 showed that DES was not effective in this regard, but it continued to be prescribed until 1971 when the Food and Drug Administration issued warnings about its use for pregnant women, citing an increase in risk of rare cancers to the children of women who took it (Adess et al. 1983). By that time, an estimated one million individuals had been exposed to the drug before birth (Konicki 1985). The effects of DES exposure are difficult to quantify scientifically, since factors such as dose, duration of exposure, and age of the mother are generally not known. Developmental stage at time of prenatal exposure is also often unknown, but undoubtedly of great importance as well (Herbst et al. 1986).

Prenatal Exposure

To date, I have been unable to find studies which show that women exposed to DES prenatally are at increased risk of breast cancer. There may be no effect, or the increase in risk may be so small it cannot be detected using our present study methods. Most of the women exposed prenatally are not yet in their postmenopausal years, so it is also possible that more time is needed for an effect to become apparent.

Exposure During Pregnancy

A 1978 study that compared the risk of breast cancer in over six hundred women who took DES and more than six hundred who did not (Bibbo et al. 1978) found no significant difference in risk between the two groups. Ages of women in the study are not given directly, but would appear to average about fifty-four. Therefore, the results apply more to premenopausal or to early postmenopausal risk than to risk in older women. Of exposed women, thirty-two developed breast cancer, compared to twenty-one of those not exposed—a difference that was not significant.

A reanalysis of the data in this study found "significantly" more diagnosed breast cancer in the group which took DES—a significance that was obtained by including only cases of cancer that could be verified by pathology review (Brian et al. 1980). Using this more stringent case definition criterion, four cases were eliminated from the control group and one from the DES group. When these small changes were made, the difference between the two groups became statistically significant. I mention the specifics here to illustrate how few changes are sometimes needed to make a result significant.

A British study of diabetics did find a significant increase in the risk of breast cancer in women who took DES (Beral and Colwell 1980). However, this study suffers from small numbers of subjects (less than one hundred in each group), and it reports on risk in diabetics only. In addition, the women were given much higher doses of DES than were used in the United States. For these reasons, the results of this study cannot be considered definitive and may not be applicable to those without diabetes or those who were given DES in the amounts typically prescribed in the United States.

A more recent study included over three thousand women who took DES and an equally large group that did not (Greenberg et al. 1984). Those who took DES were found to have a breast cancer risk 1.4 times that of the control group, a risk that was statistically significant. However, no significant difference in breast cancer mortality was found between women exposed to DES and those not exposed. When time since exposure was considered, a significant increase in risk occurred only after thirty years. Relatively few women had been exposed thirty or more years previously, so the results are not definitive. Similarly, when age at diagnosis was taken into account, significant differences in risk (2.2) were found only at ages sixty and older, when both the control and study groups were small.

Another recent study compared the risk of breast cancer in over 1,500 women who took DES during pregnancy with that of an equal number of women in the same doctors' offices who did not (Hadjimichael et al. 1984). Most of the women in this study received low doses of DES. However, no increase in risk was found with increasing dose, nor were exposed women at significantly increased risk when compared to those who were not exposed.

Brinton et al. (1986) found no significant increase in risk of breast cancer in women who took DES as a replacement hormone, even with more than ten years of use. However, the number of subjects was quite small (less than fifty in each subgroup), and subjects took DES at older ages than women exposed during pregnancy.

Many women exposed to DES either while pregnant or in utero have been profoundly affected by the experience. Those who were pregnant may feel guilt and sorrow about the medical problems some of their daughters endure. Others worry that as a result of their DES exposure they might be particularly susceptible to the effects of techniques such as mammography or to hormone replacement therapy.

Some are reassured when they realize that the radiation dose of modern-day mammograms is very low. (For a further discussion of mammography, see Chapter 7.) Some become less concerned about replacement hormones when they realize that these hormones differ in structure from DES, and of the evidence to date suggesting that women who take replacement hormones are at little or no increased risk of breast cancer up to thirty years following use.

Some remain profoundly suspicious of medications and medical interventions. They quite reasonably cite their own history and the history of others who have suffered greatly as a result of DES exposure, a hormone once considered safe. Given their experiences, they understandably ask how they can trust again, particularly when no studies exist that specifically focus on the effects of mammograms or the effects of replacement hormones on women who took DES or who were exposed in utero.

My response is to turn to the scientific method and to analyze studies now available to us. Once these studies have been thoroughly evaluated, with the numbers and methodology analyzed, I think it often becomes possible for each woman to weigh risks and benefits in making health care decisions. Unfortunately, such studies were not available for women to analyze before they were given DES; indeed, it was not usual from 1950 to 1970 for women to be consulted about medical care or asked to weigh the risks and benefits of various options. With studies more widely publicized these days, and with individuals more involved in making decisions about their own medical care, today's women are more likely to have the means to make informed decisions.

In summary, studies of women exposed to DES while pregnant generally find no increase in breast cancer risk, or find a small increase in risk that becomes significant only thirty or more years after exposure. Those exposed form a small group, so the results are not definitive. One study of women who took DES as a replacement hormone found no increase in risk to users compared to nonusers, but the sample size was small. Increased breast cancer risks to daughters exposed in utero has not been shown. Most of these daughters are still premenopausal, so future studies will be needed to determine risk of breast cancer to this group at older ages.

6

Family History and Genetics

Many misconceptions about breast cancer risk are related to family history. For example, some people assume that risk increases proportionately with the number of affected relatives, or that a propensity to increased risk skips a generation, putting women with an affected grandmother at particularly high risk. Others feel they need not be concerned about risk if only their paternal relatives were diagnosed with breast cancer. And many women think there is almost no chance they will be diagnosed with breast cancer because "no one in my family has ever had it." None of these beliefs is correct.

In the United States, 85 percent to 90 percent of the women diagnosed with breast cancer have no close relative with this disease. Therefore, in most families, breast cancer is a sudden, unexpected occurrence. When breast cancer does occur, in most cases the cause (or causes) is unknown. At the present time, there are no laboratory tests to distinguish between a woman who carries a gene or genes that significantly increase her risk of breast cancer and one who does not. In most cases, breast cancer is thought to result from an interaction of an individual's genes and the environment. That is, rarely is an individual genetically programmed to develop breast cancer. Most of us think of radiation exposure or diet as environmental factors that might cause breast cancer. However, as my geneticist colleague, Dr. David E. Anderson at the M. D. Anderson Cancer Center, notes, a factor generally classified as an environmental agent appears to have its effect on the intracellular level, and also on the genes. (See below for a further discussion of the interaction between genes and the environment.)

In many older studies, women with an affected mother or sister were found to have a two- to fourfold increase in risk of breast cancer, compared to those without such a family history (Henderson et al. 1977). It was not until the 1970s, when Dr. Anderson began to distinguish between different types of family histories, that analysis in this area became more precise. Dr. Anderson's studies identified two different types of family histories. In the first type of family, which I call Type I, breast cancer is present in a single generation—two or more sisters are affected, but their mother and daughters are not. In the second type of family (Type II), breast cancer is present in two or more generations—a grandmother and mother or a sister and mother are affected. As might be expected, Dr. Anderson found that women in Type II families have a higher risk of breast cancer than those in Type I families. Dr. Anderson also used age at diagnosis (before or after age fifty) and presence of cancer in one breast (unilateral) or both (bilateral) in analyzing risks to relatives of breast cancer patients. He observed that in some families, where the risk of breast cancer appeared to be quite high, the age at diagnosis was decreased and the occurrence of bilateral disease was increased.

To increase the likelihood that the families investigated had a greater than average genetic predisposition, Dr. Anderson included in his studies only families in which at least two close relatives had breast cancer—a mother and daughter or two sisters. He then calculated risks to over six hundred sisters and daughters of affected women. In his early studies, he found a woman's risk was influenced by the type of family history (presence of breast cancer in one generation or two), age at diagnosis (younger than or older than fifty), and laterality (unilateral or bilateral).

In these initial studies, the group at risk contained over six hundred women, but some of the subgroups were quite small. For example, there were few who had a Type II family with bilateral disease where both relatives were diagnosed after age 50. To surmount the problem of small sample size, subgroups of women were pooled. For example, risks were calculated for women who had an affected relative with unilateral breast cancer, diagnosed at age fifty or younger, regardless of family type; in a separate set of analyses, risks were calculated for women who came from a Type I family (single generation affected), whose relatives had unilateral disease, regardless of age at diagnosis.

These complex tables now form the basis for a much-enhanced risk analysis process (Anderson and Badzioch 1985). Others have also shown that women with similar appearing family histories can have very different risks (for example, Ottman et al. 1983; Schwartz et al. 1985; Claus et al. 1990). The Ottman (1983) study, which is based on women who had at least one affected first degree relative (mother, sister, or daughter), also found an increased risk of breast cancer in those having a relative with bilateral disease. In the Schwartz (1985) study, relatives of women diagnosed at age fifty-five or younger were at higher risk when their families contained two generations of affected individuals instead of one affected generation.

More recently Claus et al. (1990) studied over four thousand women with breast cancer and four thousand without the disease. Risks were calculated for those who had multiple relatives with breast cancer. Generally, their results are similar to, and complement the results of, Dr. Anderson's work, as discussed below.

Generally speaking, women who have two close relatives with unilateral breast cancer have a lifetime breast cancer risk of about 15 percent to 20 percent (Anderson and Badzioch 1985). (As you may recall, the average woman's lifetime risk is 10 percent.) The lifetime risk is about 30 percent to 50 percent for those having a relative with bilateral disease, depending on the type of family history. For women with different types of family histories, age-specific risks, in addition to lifetime risks, are available.

Dr. Anderson's latest results show that women whose sisters are diagnosed at age fifty and younger are not at greater risk of breast cancer than those whose sisters are diagnosed at older ages. The similarity in risk is probably due to the large age range considered in this analysis. This interpretation is supported by the work of Claus et al. (1990), which found that risk to the mother or sister of a woman with breast cancer increased as the decade of onset decreased. That is, women whose relative was affected in her twenties had a higher risk than those whose relative was affected in her forties.

Dr. Anderson's work is remarkable for the large number of families studied, as well as for the care taken in verifying the presence of affected individuals. He realized that the history of disease in a family is not always what relatives have been told or have believed. I have learned firsthand that family histories are not always what they seem, and so have great respect for the care Dr. Anderson has taken in verifying the presence of breast and other cancers in the families he studied. This is not common practice in most studies, since it is time-consuming and costly.

In my own practice, I routinely order medical records to verify the type of cancer in relatives who are thought to be affected. My patients help with the record collection process, which helps to reduce costs. In many cases, individuals who assumed they knew their family history quite well have learned from the medical records that they were misinformed.

In one case, I was asked to analyze the risk to a young woman whose mother and maternal aunt were both said to have had premenopausal, bilateral breast cancer. As I began the record collection process, my patient expressed some dismay at the month or so this would take. To her, it was an unnecessary delay, since she felt she had all the necessary information on her family history. I persisted with the record collection process, only to learn that in fact neither

her mother nor her aunt had been diagnosed with breast cancer. Instead, both had received multiple biopsies for benign breast disease.

In many cases, the records serve a social as well as a scientific purpose, since they help relatives of breast cancer patients to realize that they are not doomed to follow the same course. For example, one of my patients whose mother and aunt had died of breast cancer when she was a child was sure both had small lesions. The records showed the aunt had in one breast two cancers that were 4cm and 3cm in size, while her mother's breast cancer measured over 2.5cm. My patient's confidence in early detection improved immeasurably after learning the facts about her aunt's and mother's breast cancers.

Breast Cancer Risk Analysis

Many women with a family history of breast cancer benefit greatly from a formal Breast Cancer Risk Analysis. These specialized services are designed to perform the laborious and technical risk analysis and to help individuals and their families understand the significance of these risks. The process of risk analysis is often as helpful as the specific risk information transmitted, as discussed in Chapters 1 and 7. In addition to information about genetic and environmental risk factors, Breast Cancer Risk Analysis includes help in understanding cancer etiology, background information about statistics, biology, and medicine, and about how others have dealt with cancer in the family. Individuals are helped to develop surveillance programs commensurate with their levels of risk and concern. A major focus, of course, is daughters whose mothers had breast cancer at a young age and who often think their risk is much greater than it actually is. For a listing of Breast Cancer Risk Analysis Centers in the United States, see Appendix A.

Paternal History

Increased genetic susceptibility to breast cancer can be passed as easily through the father's side of the family as through the mother's. The importance of the paternal side was elegantly shown in studies in the 1950s (Macklin 1959). Unfortunately, at the present time we have no studies based on paternal history to give age-specific risks comparable to those developed for women with a maternal history of breast cancer. Dr. Anderson has found that sisters and aunts of breast cancer patients are equally likely to be affected, regardless of whether the disease is maternally or paternally derived. In a study of 115 families, sisters of men with breast cancer were found to have the same lifetime risk of breast cancer as sisters of women with this disease (D. E. Anderson, letter to author, 1990).

Multiple Cancer Risk

In most families, if there is an increased genetic predisposition to cancer, it is generally for a single site, such as the breast. However, there are families in which individuals are at increased risk of several different primary cancers. Among the more thoroughly studied families are those in which individuals are at increased risk of breast, uterine and colon cancer or breast cancer, sarcoma, brain tumors, and leukemia. In still other families, there is an increased risk of both breast and ovarian cancer.

I want to stress that the presence of several cancers in a patient's family does not invariably mean that he or she is at increased risk of cancers at several sites. In most cases, analysis will show that the risk is not increased, since the "cancer families" described above are relatively rare. However, in families where individuals are at increased risk of several cancers, it is important for family members to have this information so they can take advantage of early detection programs and thereby improve their prognosis, should a cancer arise. This is another instance in which a thorough analysis by specialists trained in Cancer Risk Analysis is warranted.

Simple or Mendelian Inheritance

In only a small proportion of families does susceptibility to breast cancer appear to be inherited in the simple, single gene (Mendelian) inheritance patterns called recessive or dominant. (The third Mendelian type, called X-linked inheritance, is less likely to play a role, and so is not included in this discussion.)

In speaking to patients about cancer and genetics, I find it useful to remind them that individuals receive two copies of each gene, one from their mother and one from their father. I explain that there are thousands of genes that make the chemicals which in turn cause our bodies to develop, grow, and function. Genes are located on the chromosomes, which can be thought of as the unclasped necklaces on which the genes are strung like beads. Human beings receive twenty-three pairs of these chromosome necklaces, with each gene normally located at only one specific place on a given necklace pair.

All human beings are thought to have some recessive genes that could cause problems to their child or themselves—if both members of a given pair of genes are damaged or missing. Instead, most individuals appear to be born with only a single copy of several different gene pairs absent or damaged. The usual or undamaged member of the pair compensates for the other.

Recessive Inheritance

If the usual, undamaged gene pair is called RR, a person with a single problem recessive gene (r) at the R position would be Rr. An Rr individual is called a carrier, and gen-

Table 6-1. Recessive Inheritance When Both Parents Are Carriers

Parents' Genotypes		Types of Children Possible
Mother	Rr	RR = usual
Father	Rr	Rr = carrier
		Rr = carrier
		rr = affected

Key: RR = usual; Rr = carrier; rr = affected.

Table 6-2. Recessive Inheritance When One Parent Is a Carrier

Parents' Genotypes		Types of Children Possible
Mother	RR	RR = usual
Father	Rr	RR = usual
		Rr = carrier
		Rr = carrier

Key: RR = usual; Rr = carrier; rr = affected.

erally shows no symptoms. An individual with two problem recessive genes at the R position would be rr, and would be symptomatic.

As Table 6-1 shows, if both parents are Rr, there is a 25 percent chance at each conception that a child will receive two r's, and so be affected. If only one parent is Rr, it is not possible for a child to inherit two r's, so none of the children will be affected (Table 6-2). In some families, breast cancer appears to be inherited in the recessive fashion just described, but until more is known about the product of the gene or genes that increase risk of breast cancer, it is difficult to do more than mention this type of inheritance as a possibility in some families. (However, see the discussion of Knudson's two hit theory in the Interaction Between Genes and Environment section and the Oncogene section below.)

Table 6-3. Dominant Inheritance When One Parent Has Problem Gene

Parents' Genotypes		Types of Children Possible
Mother	Dd	Dd = usually affected
Father	dd	Dd = usually affected
		dd = not affected
		dd = not affected

Key: dd = usual; Dd = problem gene present, usually affected.

Dominant Inheritance

Dominant inheritance differs from recessive in that the effect of a problem gene is generally felt when only a single copy is present. The effects of a dominant gene can usually be traced over several generations. In writing about dominant inheritance, the pattern is reversed from that of recessive: the usual, undamaged gene is written in lower case (d), and the problem gene is written in upper case (D). An individual who has one copy of the problem gene (Dd) almost always shows the effects of it. As can be seen in Table 6-3, those with a dominant gene have a 50 percent chance of passing the gene on each time a child is conceived.

In some families, an increased susceptibility to breast cancer appears to be inherited in dominant fashion (Lynch 1981). Geneticists are learning that a disease may appear to be inherited as a dominant clinically, but on the molecular level the disease is due to an absence or change in both copies of a gene pair, as in recessive inheritance (Murphree and Benedict 1984). Therefore, until there is a reliable way to determine individuals who carry a specific gene or genes that increase susceptibility to breast cancer, it will be most difficult to be definitive about the presence of either dominant or recessive genes in families. (See the section on gene probes below for a discussion of some of the more recent advances in this area.) Even when susceptibility to breast cancer appears to be inherited in dominant fashion, most women in these families have a less than 50 percent lifetime risk of breast cancer. Environmental and other factors such as the action of other genes may decrease the risk.

Interaction Between Genes and Environment

Most cases of breast cancer are thought to be due not to a single dominant gene, nor to a pair of recessively inherited genes, but to an interaction between several of a woman's genes and the environment. A model of this interaction is shown in Figure 6-1 and demonstrates that, with an increase in genetic susceptibility (horizontal axis), less environmental input (vertical axis) is needed to bring about a given disease. The reverse is also true. Individuals probably differ in their genetic sensitivity to various environmental agents.

The declining incidence of stomach cancer in the United States in the last fifty years provides an example of the interaction between genes and the environment. It is unlikely that the genetic predisposition of the population as a whole has greatly changed in such a short time. Instead, it appears that as better food preservation techniques have become available, the U.S. consumption of highly pickled, salted, and smoked foods has decreased. With the reduction of these environmental factors, the incidence of stomach cancer has decreased.

Note that in Figure 6-1 the environmental factors are called *insults*. This term is used in deference to Dr. Alfred Knudson's two hit theory regarding the origin of cancer (Knudson 1971). According to this theory, a cell can be changed or *hit* by an environmental factor, thereby producing a genetic change in the cell. When the cell divides, this change is passed on to all of its daughter cells, which in turn, pass the change on to their daughter cells. Therefore, as a person gets older, the number of changed cells increases. If

Figure 6-1. Interaction of Genes and Environment

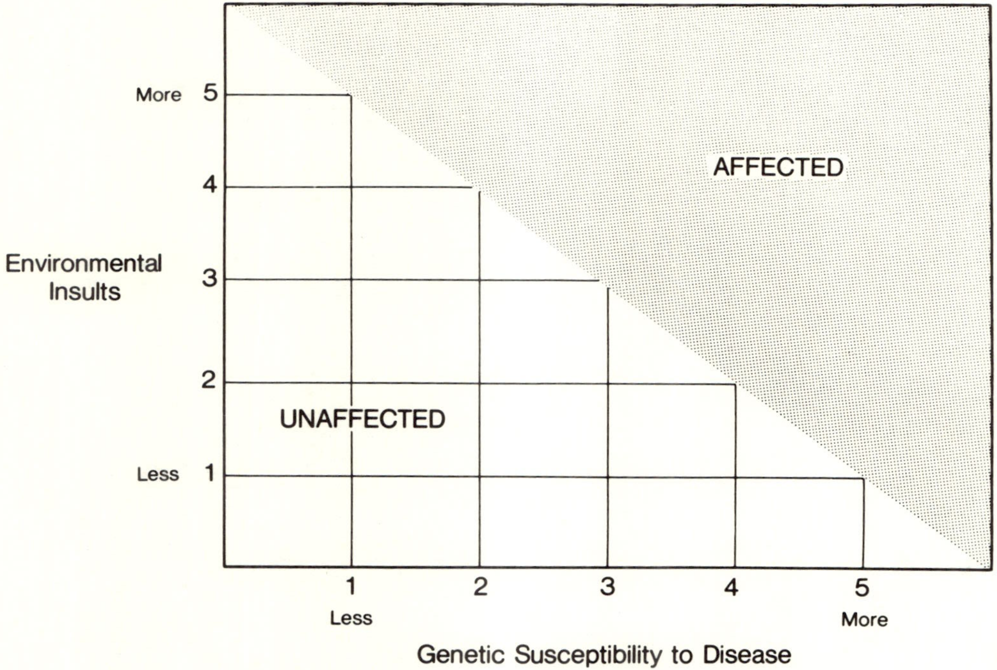

Source: From Kelly, P. T., 1983, "Genetic Counseling with the Cancer Patient's Family," *Current Problems in Cancer* 7 (12):29, fig. 1. Reprinted by permission of the copyright owner, Yearbook Medical Publishers, Inc., Chicago.

a changed cell is hit by another environmental agent, it can, in turn, be transformed to become a cancer cell. Because it takes time for a cell to receive two hits, individuals are more likely to develop cancer as they age. Knudson's theory has recently been found to apply to several rare cancers in children that are inherited in simple, single gene fashion, including retinoblastoma (Knudson 1986). To date, the theory appears to apply to the more frequent cancers found in adults as well.

Gene Probes or Restriction Fragment Length Polymorphisms (RFLP)

In the past few years, technological breakthroughs have occurred that will probably make it possible in the future to test individuals for their genetic sensitivities to many environmental substances, as well as to detect which members of a family carry an increased genetic susceptibility to diseases such as breast cancer. A new test, called the Restriction Fragment Length Polymorphism test (RFLP, or gene probe), uses normal genetic variations as markers to determine who is or is not a carrier for various problem genes whose approximate, but not precise, location may be known or whose gene product is unknown. This test is already being used to detect carriers of genes for diseases such as Duchenne muscular dystrophy and polyposis colon cancer. The use of the RFLP test in detecting those at increased susceptibility to many other diseases will no doubt follow shortly.

The RFLP test works by taking advantage of the many normal gene variations found along all of the chromosomes. Health professionals are accustomed to these normal variants in considering the ABO blood group, where different individuals in the same family can be, for example, AO, AA, or AB. The gene probe test makes use of similar normal genetic variations at other specific locations on the chromosomes. Special enzymes (restriction enzymes) are used to cut or slice a chromosome only at the location of specific normal gene

Figure 6-2. Example of How RFLP Test Might Detect Increased Genetic Susceptibility to Breast Cancer in Future

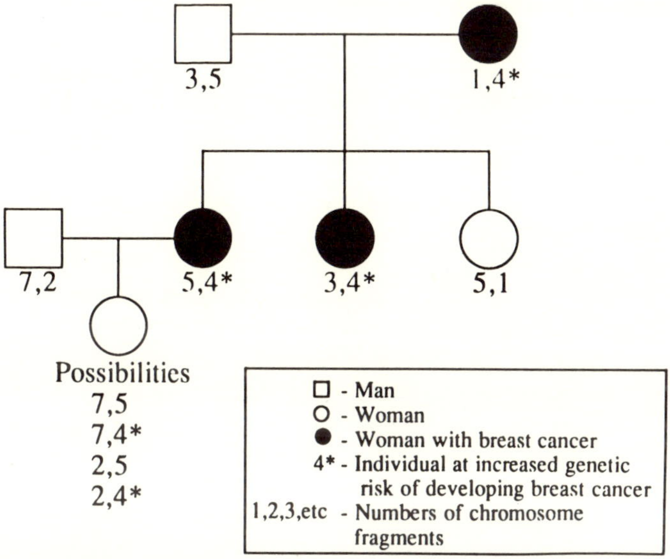

variations. Individuals who have a particular genetic variation on both members of a chromosome pair will have both chromosomes cut at that location, while those who have the variation on neither chromosome will have neither cut. A person who has the variant on one chromosome of a chromosome pair will have only that chromosome cut. Each of these individuals will produce a different pattern of chromosome pieces or fragments. The actual testing method is more complex, but essentially makes use of different fragments as markers for the presence of a problem gene.

Colleagues in the field tell me they believe a test for some of the more common cancers, such as breast cancer, are three to five years away. When these tests are available, it may be possible to determine individual susceptibilities to breast cancer, as shown in Figure 6-2. I find it useful to inform patients of new developments such as these, even if they cannot yet be of use to them or their families; information of such advances can provide much needed hope. In addition, some families may wish to store or bank DNA of certain elderly or ill relatives for possible future RFLP testing. To see if your patients are eligible for such a program, you may wish to contact the Breast Cancer Risk Analysis Service in your area (see Appendix A).

Oncogenes

In explaining oncogenes to patients, I find it useful to first remind them that humans carry a virtually complete genetic makeup in almost all cells. Regulator genes, as well as other control mechanisms, help cells to remember their specialized roles. As an example, I tell them, a skin cell must be regulated to keep the genes for corneal formation from being expressed in the skin.

I then explain that oncogenes are changed forms of normal genes that control growth and development, called proto-oncogenes. By 1989, over fifty oncogenes had been detected (Taylor 1989). When a proto-oncogene is lost or damaged, cell regulation is disturbed. The unregulated growth that occurs is called cancer.

SUMMARY

In the last few years, new techniques have been developed that may make it possible to determine whether an individual is at increased risk of developing a cancer. Until these tests are available, we will continue to make use of family history analyses and risk tables, which show that not all women with a family history of breast cancer have the same risk. Instead, a woman's risk appears to be influenced by the type of family history, laterality, and, in some families, by the age at which a woman's relatives were affected.

In most individuals, breast cancer appears to be brought about by an interaction between genes and the environment, not just by the action of a single gene. Genetic susceptibility to breast cancer is transmitted as easily through the father's side of the family as through the mother's. In some rare families, individuals are at an increased genetic risk of developing several different types of cancers.

A new test called Restriction Fragment Length Polymorphism (RFLP, or gene probe) has made it possible to use normal variations between individuals to detect those with increased genetic susceptibility to disease. Scientists are now trying to develop such a test for breast and other cancers.

(As this book went to press, evidence was published of a gene located on chromosome 17 that is associated with an increased risk of breast cancer in some families [J. M. Hall, M. K. Lee, B. Newman, et al. 1990. "Linkage of Early-Onset Familial Breast Cancer to Chromosome 17921." *Science* 250: 1684–89.])

7

Helping Patients with a Breast Concern

Patients today have often read and heard conflicting advice about effective breast health care. Many wonder if their own personal circumstances necessitate a modification of the generally recommended guidelines. Some need help feeling comfortable with advice offered by health professionals, even those whom they trust. The emotional words of one patient illustrate the dilemma faced by many patients these days:

> How do I decide what to do? It's not that I don't trust my doctor. I do! I do! It's just that I don't know what to make of all the different advice I'm getting from him and from what I've read.

Defining Prudent Breast Health Care

This chapter focuses on information and counseling techniques useful in helping patients achieve reasonable breast health care and treatments. Given the great concern about breast cancer in the United States today, it is not surprising that thoughts about breast health care can generate highly emotional reactions even in women who have no symptoms. Patients often ask anxiously what they should do to establish a reasonable breast health care program. They have heard, of course, of breast self-examinations, mammograms, and examinations by a health professional, but wonder about the frequency and accuracy of these procedures, and whether they actually make a difference in a woman's life expectancy if a breast cancer should be found.

With all the publicity about the value of early detection, women often ask why the death rate due to breast cancer has not changed significantly in recent years (see Figure 7-1). Many worry that the rather constant death rate is an indication that early detection may not be as effective as claimed. Actually, the scientific evidence shows that early detection of breast cancer does improve prognosis but, to date, many women in the United States have not had this benefit. For example, tumor size is a critical determinant of survival. In the United States, in 1987, the average invasive breast cancer measured 25mm (1 inch) in size at the time of diagnosis. Half of breast cancers 25mm in size have already metastasized to local lymph nodes (Donegan and Spratt 1979), but at the 5mm size, the chance of metastasis is 20 percent or less, depending on the type of breast cancer (Fisher et al. 1969). Generally speaking, the smaller a breast cancer, the less likely it is to have metastasized and the better the prognosis (Yang et al. 1987). Until the average size of breast cancers diagnosed in the United States is reduced to less than 10mm, we will probably not see a significant decline in the death rate due to this disease. This is not a failure of early detection methods, but of bringing these methods within the reach of all American women.

Mammography

A Swedish study, which compared over 134,000 women who did and did not receive regular mammograms over a six to seven year period, found that screened women were significantly more likely to be diagnosed with smaller breast cancers than were those who did not receive regular mammograms (Tabar et al. 1985). Breast cancer death rates were signifi-

Figure 7-1. Cancer Death Rates in U.S. Women, 1930–1985

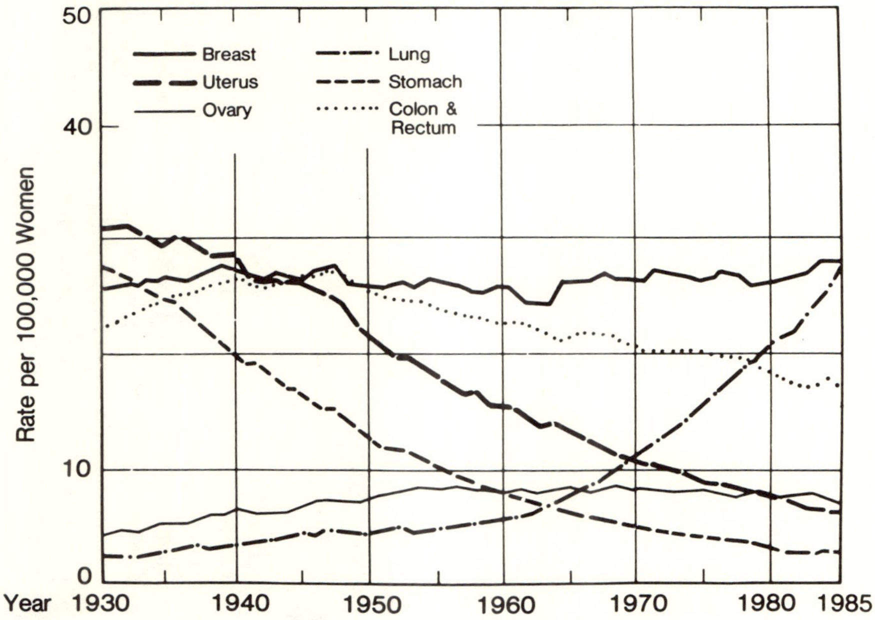

Source: Adapted from U.S. National Center for Health Statistics and U.S. Bureau of the Census, 1989, as cited in "Cancer Death Rate in Women, 1930–1985," *Ca—A Cancer Journal for Clinicians* 39 (1989):10. Copyright by the American Cancer Society, Inc., and *Ca—A Cancer Journal for Clinicians*.

cantly reduced (relative risk of 0.6) in women aged fifty to seventy-four who received regular mammograms. No significant reduction in death rate was seen in screened women aged forty to forty-nine, but fewer than twenty deaths occurred in either the study or control groups of women this age. Larger numbers will be needed to show a benefit to this group.

In another study of over 62,000 U.S. women, the 31,000 who were carefully followed with both mammograms and breast examinations by a physician had a 22 percent reduction in deaths due to breast cancer compared to those who were not regularly followed in this way (Habbema et al. 1986). Reductions in mortality were found for all age groups, but unlike the screened group as a whole, the differences by age were not statistically significant. Recent analyses of these data show a true reduction in those who died of breast cancer, not merely a longer life among women diagnosed at an earlier stage (Shapiro 1989). Still another study found a 30 percent increase in survival among women followed closely with mammograms and breast examinations (Letton and Mason 1986). It now seems clear that early detection techniques can lead to an improved prognosis.

Most women have heard that mammograms can detect breast cancer at early stages. Many question how often they need this procedure, how old they should be at the time of their initial mammogram, and what effects the radiation they receive might have on their health over time. In 1989, a number of physician organizations joined with the American Cancer Society to endorse the following mammography recommendations: for asymptomatic women, a baseline mammogram between the ages of thirty-five and forty, with mammograms every year or two from age forty to forty-nine. Women age fifty and older are advised to have annual mammograms. Those with a family history of breast cancer or who are thought to be at increased risk for other reasons are advised to start a baseline mammogram at earlier ages, between thirty and thirty-five, and may also be advised to obtain mammograms at more frequent intervals.

Breast cancers detected by mammography are smaller than those found by palpation and are less likely to have spread to lymph nodes. These are the earliest and most curable lesions. In fact, mammograms can successfully find breast cancers too small to be felt by the most adept physical examination (Margolin and Lagios 1986). Most studies report that 30 percent to 40 percent of all breast cancers can be detected by mammography alone. Over the years, the ability to detect small breast cancers by mammography has improved. In 1988, at Children's Hospital in San Francisco, 72 percent of all breast cancers detected were found using mammography alone (F. Margolin, discussion with author, 1990).

When patients question the safety of mammograms, I tell them the dose of radiation they receive is about 0.2 rads, the equivalent of several trips across the country by jet (cosmic rays are more intense at higher altitudes), or the equivalent of living for a year in an area such as Denver, Colorado, where the background radiation is particularly high. When patients realize that the X-ray dose from modern mammograms is this small, and are helped to compare these small risks with the large benefits, they tend to feel more comfortable and are more likely to make use of this early detection technique.

In helping patients to choose where they will obtain mammograms, you may want to learn the following about mammography at the institutions in your area: the usual radiation dose per exposure (less than 1 rad), the number of mammograms performed (more than ten a day), and quality assurance procedures for monitoring accuracy of technologist positioning and physician interpretation. A machine dedicated to mammography alone is mandatory. A film processor dedicated to mammography is also preferable. Obviously, an institution or group with more experience, that specializes in breast health care, and that has up-to-date equipment and a well-trained staff is preferable to one without these features. In 1987, the American College of Radiology began a voluntary accreditation program for mammography facilities, providing another source for you to evaluate any mammographic facility. In most states, the department of health and human services oversees the registration and inspection of mammographic equipment, and can be called upon to help evaluate the safety of mammography in a community.

Breast Self-examinations

Effective breast health care is based on both physical breast examinations and mammograms, with neither being a replacement for the other. About 75 percent of all breast cancers are found by women themselves (Nemoto et al. 1982), suggesting that with regular practice, this complementary method could help more women find smaller breast cancers at an earlier stage. Many women are not aware that even with the best mammographic techniques currently available, 10 percent or more of breast cancers, regardless of size, may be invisible on mammograms (Margolin and Lagios 1986). For this reason, examinations by a health professional and breast self-examinations (BSE) continue to be important. In my experience, it is not sufficient to tell women they must, or should, practice breast self-examination. Instead, they need to be taught the procedure in a thoughtful, careful manner that enables them to gain the self-confidence needed to become proficient at a new skill.

Breast Examinations by Health Professionals

Patients often ask how they can be sure they are receiving quality breast examinations from their physician or nurse. Many find their confidence in the examination is enhanced if the elements composing a thorough breast examination are summarized by the health professional—that is, a quality breast examination involves raising hands over the head for visual inspection, as well as methodical palpation of the breast while the patient is sitting and lying down. This expenditure of time appears to be worthwhile, since physicians' abilities to detect abnormal lumps appear to be directly related to the time taken to perform the exam (Fletcher et al.

1985). In 1989, the American Cancer Society and physician organizations recommended that women age forty and older have a yearly physical breast examination. Those with a family history or other concern may, of course, find it useful to have an examination by a health professional every four to six months.

Some women, particularly those who have a strong family history of cancer or who have benign breast disease, say they find it almost impossible to examine their own breasts:

> Any time I examine myself I have to face the question of whether there's something going on and it's almost like I can't even ask myself that question. So I may examine myself and I'll feel something and I'll get anxious and say to myself, well I know I'm anxious anyway, so how do I know what I am really feeling in my breast?

Women with increased concerns certainly warrant more frequent and careful follow-up by health professionals than those who have no such concerns or fears.

Many patients say their doctor or nurse does not leave enough time for them to ask questions, or that they remember important questions only after the visit. (For the sake of brevity, the terms physician or doctor are used in the following discussion. Many nurses also examine breasts, of course.) I suggest that patients write down their questions as they are identified in my office and at home, think about them before their doctor's visit, *and tell the doctor's office when making the appointment to schedule extra time for discussion and questions.* Most patients don't realize, unless instructed, that the physician's office needs to know about the time they need in advance so the physician is not rushed.

Such an approach may prevent the agony my patient Sharon endured when she found a breast lump. She did not tell her doctor about it during a routine visit because she thought she had already taken up enough of his time. Fortunately for Sharon, a friend insisted she return to the doctor a week later and show him the lump. When removed, it was found to be a small breast cancer, treated with lumpectomy and radiation therapy, and associated with an excellent prognosis. Not all women are this fortunate. I have seen many over the years who waited months to years in reporting a breast lump, with disastrous results.

Unfortunately, women who feel they are at increased risk may be particularly reluctant to schedule more frequent physician examinations, for fear they will be called hypochondriacs. Many speak of feeling caught between the extremes:

> You start feeling you are making a mountain out of a molehill or that things are being withheld from you. You vacillate between the two.

> Doctors either tell you that you're too young, you're imagining things, or you face this drastic thing of having both breasts removed.

Information and help in formulating a breast health program can help to assuage feelings such as these and also guide women toward safer health practices.

Guidelines

The following guidelines have helped my patients with a breast lump, change, or concern to better plan, prepare, and work cooperatively with their physicians. They are presented here for you to use in helping your patients:

- Try not to panic. Remember that most breast changes are found to be benign.
- Schedule an appointment with your doctor as soon as possible, but don't worry about a delay of a few days.
- Take a friend or relative with you to doctors' visits, especially those in which treatment will be discussed.
- If the doctor asks you to return in a month, do so, even if a mammogram finds no evidence of breast cancer, and you think the worrisome area is no longer present.

- If a single, dominant, discrete lump or distinctive area persists in your breast more than a month, and a doctor suggests following it over time, consider seeking a second opinion from another physician. Choose, for your consultation, a breast specialist outside the medical community of the first. Many doctors feel that an isolated breast lump or changed area that persists should be removed.
- If you have a breast change, and your doctor has not recommended a mammogram, ask why not. This is another time you might consider obtaining a second opinion, especially if you are over thirty years of age.
- If a mammogram shows a change or a suspicious area, but you and your doctor cannot feel a lump, remember that most physicians recommend a biopsy at such times. If your physician does not, a second medical opinion may be warranted.
- Let your doctor know if his or her advice or treatment plan is unclear. It is not your job to ease the doctor's busy schedule by taking less time. Instead, your job is to learn enough to make an informed decision.
- Tell your friends and relatives what you understand the specifics of your diagnosis, treatment, or follow-up to be. If you find you can't explain it to them, ask the doctor to explain the issues to you again.

For the sake of brevity, I have not mentioned needle biopsies in the above guidelines. Obviously, in some cases, as when a cyst is suspected, a needle biopsy will be performed that might obviate the need for excisional biopsy. Many centers are also performing fine-needle aspiration for any palpable findings to more accurately assess the index of suspicion of a breast lesion.

Second Opinions

These days, many women are aware of the value of a second medical opinion, and so may consult several surgeons once a breast lesion is detected or a breast cancer diagnosed. After a diagnosis of breast cancer, I find my patients are increasingly seeking opinions from a radiation oncologist as well. They realize that different specialists have different perspectives, and until their case has been evaluated by a radiation oncologist, they have not yet sufficiently explored all options. Many also consult a medical oncologist to discuss the advisability of chemotherapy or hormonal treatments. Plastic surgeons are also increasingly involved in the primary treatment if total mastectomy is indicated and immediate reconstruction is feasible and desireable.

The importance of a second pathology opinion is not as yet generally recognized. The absence of this consultation is unfortunate since, as I tell my patients, pathology is like an architect's plan: it distinguishes a castle from a cottage, even though both are buildings. Or, as a pathologist colleague of mine said, "Some breast cancers behave like lap dogs and others like pit bulls." It is the pathologist's job to translate what he or she sees under the microscope so that the health professional and patient can understand the particular features of the benign and/or malignant cells found.

In the past, a pathologist's analysis of breast biopsy material focused primarily on the presence or absence of invasive disease. These days, with knowledge of benign breast cells that can mimic invasion, with the concern that invasive cells can be overlooked if not all of the biopsy material is examined, and with a growing appreciation that different types of breast cancer warrant different treatments, the focus of pathology has broadened in some institutions to provide a more accurate description of the breast cells, whether benign or malignant (for example, size, grade, or aggressiveness are now more likely to be included in a pathology report). The correlation between the mammogram and the biopsied tissue is especially critical when the sole means of detection has been mammographic.

The tremendous importance of a second pathology opinion was made clear to me several years ago, as I discussed a distressing breast cancer with Susan, the mother of three young children. Two and a half months after the birth of her last child, she felt a lump in her breast which proved to be about 5cm in diameter and was diagnosed as invasive breast cancer. By the time I saw Susan, she and her husband had sought opinions from several surgeons, all of whom recommended immediate mastectomy, followed by radiation therapy. She had seen a medical oncologist, who recommended immediate chemotherapy, followed by mastectomy. While I was talking to Susan, the pathologist to whom I had sent her slides for review called to say that invasive breast cancer did not comprise 5cm of the lesion, but was instead so small he called it microinvasive. The initial pathologist had failed to distinguish between areas of duct carcinoma in situ and invasion. (For a discussion of the difference between invasive and in situ breast cancers see Chapter 3).

The surgeons and medical oncologist whom Susan saw had access to only the initial pathology report when they gave their opinions, and so had been led to believe that the entire lesion was composed of invasive cells. As a result of the pathology review, Susan's doctors realized her prognosis was much improved. All agreed that she did not need either chemotherapy or a mastectomy. Following her lumpectomy and axillary lymph node dissection, in which no positive nodes were found, she received six weeks of radiation therapy. As expected, she has had no recurrence of her cancer.

In summary, effective breast health care consists of mammograms, breast self-examinations, and examinations by a health professional. Mammograms can detect small breast cancers that cannot be palpated, but cannot detect all breast cancers, making physical breast examinations an essential component of early detection. Women often find that one-on-one teaching of breast self-examination increases confidence in their own abilities to practice it. Patients who are not comfortable with breast self-examination may benefit from more frequent and regular examinations by a health professional who specializes in breast health care. Women who receive regular follow-up care for their breasts have significantly improved prognoses compared to those who do not. The smaller a breast cancer, the less likely it has spread, and the better the prognosis.

Health professionals can provide great assistance to patients with breast problems or concerns by helping them to formulate new questions, providing a safe place in which they can sort out their thoughts and feelings, helping them to integrate the information they have received, discussing ramifications of different treatment options, and encouraging second opinions.

Patients often need encouragement to thoroughly explore options before making treatment decisions. This generally involves a pathology review and consultations with a medical oncologist, a radiation oncologist, as well as a surgeon and plastic surgeon. Second opinions are generally quite useful. Only when a woman is given the time and opportunity to understand the information she has been given can her decisions be considered informed.

Counseling and Health Education Techniques

Counseling and health education techniques can be useful in helping patients who are confused or frightened to formulate new questions and to better understand ramifications of the information they are given. With patients who have a breast concern, these techniques take into account each person's reactions to illness in general and breast cancer specifically. Instead of ignoring emotional reactions, decrying their existence, or waiting for them to pass before attempting to convey information, I find the counseling approach most useful that fully accepts the presence of emotion. In fact, by identifying a patient's reactions to breast cancer and breast cancer risk during the first visit, communication is often greatly facilitated.

Some health professionals worry that if patients are encouraged to talk about fears and concerns while in the process of making decisions, a floodgate of emotions might be released with potentially harmful consequences. Proponents of this school of thought either defer a discussion or even acknowledgment of emotions until the informational issues have been covered, or ignore emotions altogether. As will be discussed later, unacknowledged emotional reactions can act as barriers that prevent a patient from understanding even carefully presented information.

Individuals generally obtain relief and release when they are given an opportunity to discuss their feelings, and are encouraged to acknowledge emotions that are a normal outgrowth of their life experiences. Patients who express emotions are often able to focus more effectively on information than are those who do not. Also, learning about an individual's feelings and experiences helps health professionals to determine how to effectively present information to that person.

In the course of Breast Cancer Risk Analysis, some individuals learn their risk of this disease is quite high, or is higher than they had thought. In such cases, patient self-image may change from being a healthy to a sick person or from being a so-called normal person to one who is likely to be a carrier of increased genetic susceptibility to cancer. Such changes in self-image may arouse feelings of anger, fear, or resistance. Therefore, health professionals must be able to deal with the emotions that bad news or the recognition of increased risk can bring.

Perhaps less generally recognized is the change in self-image that can occur when individuals are given good news. Those who are told their risk is lower than they had thought, or who learn they are not at increased risk of cancer, may also suffer feelings of disorientation. It is not unusual for those who receive good news to report several weeks later that they have forgotten the information they were given, or that they have thought of additional risk factors or new circumstances that might increase their risk. These individuals may need follow-up visits in which their new concerns are resolved and information is reviewed.

Assessing Emotional Reactions

Quite normal emotional reactions to even the thought of breast cancer can act as barriers to effective communication. Some reactions specific to women whose mothers had breast cancer are discussed in Chapter 1. Others relevant to concerned women in general are briefly mentioned here. This discussion is by no means intended to be inclusive or definitive; instead, it is a sampling of some of the more frequent strong reactions that can hinder communication.

Denial Some women are so frightened about breast cancer that they deny they have any risk at all. As a result of denial, a woman may not make use of early detection procedures or may even delay seeking a physician's care when obvious symptoms arise. By acknowledging risk, some believe they would be opening the door to so much fear, anxiety, and depression that they would be unable to go on with their lives in a constructive manner. Unfortunately, the energy required to maintain denial may result in lethargy, a pessimistic outlook, and a general inability to enjoy life.

Fear Fear is, of course, closely linked to denial; individuals frequently deny because they are afraid. Many women have exaggerated fears about their risk of breast cancer, due, in part, to past experiences with this disease and to misinformation. Information about breast cancer etiology, risk, new treatments, and the value of early detection can often do much to allay such fears.

Some women are subject to sudden waves of fear that are almost incapacitating, even if no symptoms are present. For example, one woman became extremely anxious after watching a television program on early detection of breast cancer. While people are in a state of fear, they generally hear or absorb little information. They may even incorrectly interpret a health professional's demeanor or tone of voice and assume the worst.

Some women say they fear mastectomy more than breast

cancer, and express very strong feelings about this surgery and the physicians who perform it:

> I feel hatred toward the doctor who would do a mastectomy, even though it would keep me alive.
>
> I don't believe butchering a person for life is good. You must leave something to build on.
>
> It's not good to get up in the morning and see half a person—or for a husband to see half a person. It's better to be dead.

Others feel they could deal with the loss of a breast quite well. To them, the effects of chemotherapy or the uncertainty associated with a cancer diagnosis are more frightening to contemplate than mastectomy. Until the health professional understands what a woman's breasts and the term breast cancer mean to her, it is unlikely that effective communication will occur. For example, in speaking about breast cancer, the health professional may mean a minimal breast cancer with a 95 percent to 99 percent survival to ten years. The patient, on the other hand, may think of breast cancer as inevitably leading to mastectomy followed by almost certain death.

Anger Those who have seen cancer in a friend or relative may feel angry about the fear, pain, and even death their loved ones have suffered, as well as the fear and loss they themselves have endured. As a result, some have a hostile manner even while seeking help. This hostility is often defused when they learn that many women with similar experiences feel angry, since anger is a normal human reaction to some of life's difficult experiences. By acknowledging and discussing anger, many patients achieve a better understanding and appreciation of the difficult times they, their friend, or their relative endured in dealing with breast cancer.

Embarrassment Women often speak of their reluctance to ask health professionals for more frequent checkups, for help in learning how to examine their own breasts, or even for the health professional's reasons for suggesting or not suggesting a mammogram or biopsy. They are embarrassed by their intense concern and worry the health professional will think they are hypochondriacs. Some tell me they waited years for a doctor to ask if they were concerned or wanted a breast examination. Women who are too embarrassed to seek repeat breast examinations from a single health professional may schedule visits with several different specialists over the year—the allergist, gynecologist, internist, and others. Even then they may not ask for a breast examination, but wait for the doctor or nurse to suggest it.

Low Self-esteem Individuals with low self-esteem have a negative perception of themselves that can lead to depression, denial, fear, guilt, and embarrassment. They may suffer from a distortion of perception that can result in a misinterpretation of the information they are given. For example, low self-esteem may lead an individual to think that even a low risk means she is doomed to develop breast cancer ("No matter what the odds, bad things always happen to me.") As a result of low self-esteem, some women believe they lack the intelligence to be able to absorb information and so neither seek it nor pay attention when it is given. Others feel they are not worthy of information or of good medical care. These persons often will not ask questions about their deepest concerns or pursue issues that are troubling them, unless helped to do so by a health professional.

Stress Individuals' emotional reactions to cancer, as well as the effort required to care for those with breast cancer, can cause a great deal of stress. It is not unusual for women with affected friends and relatives to suffer from ulcers, aching backs and necks, teeth grinding, and nightmares. For many, the process of learning more about breast cancer and their own risks, and determining the best breast health program for themselves, affords great relief. In some cases, of course, information and health planning are not sufficient. Some may need information about, and access to, more structured stress-reduction techniques, such as biofeedback, meditation, and psychological counseling.

Acknowledging Social and Emotional Ramifications

Women who have a friend or relative with breast cancer are likely to be more emotional about this disease than those who lack firsthand experience. However, even those who don't know someone personally may be influenced by what they hear of another's experience and incorrectly assume that person's experiences represent normal progression of the disease. Health professionals can be of great help in educating patients so their views of prognosis following a breast cancer diagnosis are kept up to date.

Most friends and relatives of breast cancer patients need an opportunity to discuss their experiences with or reactions to cancer and to express their feelings about them. Unfortunately, many have never had an opportunity to do this in a comprehensive manner. I encourage patients to tell their stories. Whatever their life experiences, patients need help in understanding more clearly the origins of their concerns, which often become more clear as they talk. Many have been so busy coping with the social and emotional consequences of their experiences that they have failed to appreciate how difficult the time has been for them.

Patients frequently say their reactions to breast cancer in a friend or relative have been extreme, out of control, or inexplicable, leading some to doubt their stability, ability to make decisions, or ability to cope. On the one hand, women speak cogently of the fears breast cancer engenders. On the other, they may be truly frightened by the intensity of these emotions. Health professionals can do much to help such patients re-establish equilibrium by pointing out that it is natural and healthy to be affected by strong feelings. I often say, when a woman apologizes for crying, "If you don't cry at a time like this, what are you saving the tears for?"

Information and Counseling

Two intricate and important tasks—information and counseling—are needed to help women understand and deal with their concerns about breast cancer and its risk. In view of the complexity involved, care must be taken to keep the overall objectives in view. For example, information should not be neglected in favor of an exploration of emotional and social aspects. Conversely, if emotional barriers to communication are not carefully identified, a great deal of time may be spent giving information that is either not relevant to, or is not fully understood by, that patient.

Problems can arise from the perceived or real power and influence of the health professional. In some cases, this influence may be due to transference—the health professional is imbued with characteristics similar to those of a parent or other authority figure in the patient's life. In other instances, the health professional has great influence because the visits occur during a crisis period in the patient's life. Women who have a breast concern are often somewhat anxious and upset. Their family systems and personal lives may be disrupted due to fear, leading some to become temporarily more dependent and unrealistic. Unless this issue is recognized from the outset, the patient may develop an attachment to a health professional that can interfere with the educational and counseling process.

There are several ways to keep patients from idealizing the health professional to an unrealistic extent. One is to see both members of a couple together, and to encourage those who are not part of a couple to bring a friend or relative to their visits. If a woman must always come alone to her visits, it is up to the health professional to make the missing person's presence felt. This can be done by asking what the spouse, friend, or other relative thinks or might think about the various issues that arise.

Epilogue: Breast Cancer Risk Analysis Today and in the Future

Patients often ask why more is not known about breast cancer etiology and risk, or why better treatments for breast cancer are not available. My response is to tell them about all that has been accomplished in the last few years, including:

- Development of the gene probe (RFLP) test, which will probably make it possible in the next few years to determine individuals at increased genetic risk of breast cancer
- Increased understanding of the origins of cancer, specifically research on oncogenes and regulator genes
- Improvements in early detection techniques, such as mammograms, which have already significantly reduced the death rate in those regularly screened
- Increased use of breast conserving methods in the treatment of breast cancer
- Growing acknowledgment that women with a breast concern need time to seek information about treatment options
- Acknowledgment that improved treatment modalities and increased options may be available if time is taken to obtain specific information about the pathology of a breast lesion

- Increased understanding of the heterogeneity of benign breast disease
- Growing information about in situ breast cancers and the treatment options available for them
- Acceptance of second opinions for women with a breast concern

Some of the important advances have been social. Women are now less likely to feel they should suffer in silence or should live with fear and concern about their breast health. Special centers for breast health care are springing up across the country. In June 1989, I saw a list of over one hundred fifty such centers (see National Consortium of Breast Centers in Appendix B).

Even more recent are Breast Cancer Risk Analysis services, which are designed to provide extensive information about a woman's risk, background information about the etiology of breast cancer and other factors, and information about others' reactions in a similar situation. In addition, such services help to guide patients toward appropriate breast health care and provide much needed help in dealing with the social and psychological effects of this disease on the individual and family (see Appendix A).

Over the years, I have found that women and their families, when given information and the time to absorb it, make health and medical care decisions that are right for them. Information about the genetic and environmental causes of breast cancer, as well as the social ramifications of breast cancer, helps patients with a breast concern and their families to better cope with this disease and to live lives free of unnecessary anxiety.

Appendix A: Breast Cancer Risk Analysis Services

Breast Evaluation Center
Memorial Medical Center of Long Beach
2880 Atlantic Avenue, Suite 100
Long Beach, California 90806
(213) 595-3838

Breast Health Center
Children's Hospital of San Francisco
3700 California Street
San Francisco, California 94118
(415) 750-6420

Komen Alliance Clinical Breast Center
Charles A. Sammons Cancer Center
Baylor University Medical Center
3500 Gaston Avenue
Dallas, Texas 75246
(214) 820-6975
(800) 4-BAYLOR

Appendix B: Patient Education Resources

American Cancer Society National Headquarters (also many local chapters)
15999 Clifton Road NE
Atlanta, Georgia 30329
(800) 227-2345

Mammatech Corporation (breast self-examination training and materials)
900 Northwest 8th Avenue
Gainesville, Florida 32601
(800) 626-2273

National Alliance of Breast Cancer Organizations
1180 Avenue of the Americas, second floor
New York, New York 10036
(212) 719-0154

National Cancer Institute (informative booklets)
Public Inquiry Section, Office of Cancer Communications
National Cancer Institute
Building 31, Room 10A 24
Bethesda, Maryland 20892
(800) 4-CANCER

National Consortium of Breast Centers
Attn: Barbara Rabinowitz, R.N., M.S.W., A.C.S.W.
Comprehensive Breast Center
UMDNJ—Robert Wood Johnson Medical School
One Robert Wood Johnson Place, CN19
New Brunswick, New Jersey 08903
(201) 937-7868

Y-ME National Organization for Breast Cancer Information and Support
18220 Harwood Avenue
Homewood, Illinois 60430
(800) 221-2141

Appendix C: Further Reading

American Cancer Society. June 1990. *A New Approach—The 7 P's for BSE*. Pamphlet no. 6438.39.

Donegan, W. L., and Spratt, J. S. 1989. *Cancer of the Breast*. Philadelphia: W. B. Saunders.

Haagensen, C. D. 1986. *Diseases of the Breast*. Philadelphia: W. B. Saunders.

Haagensen, C. D., M. S. Bodian, and D. E. Haagensen. 1981. *Breast Carcinoma Risk and Detection*. Philadelphia: W. B. Saunders.

Harris, J. R., S. Hellman, I. C. Henderson, et al., eds. 1987. *Breast Diseases*. Philadelphia: J. B. Lippincott.

Love, S. M. 1990. *Dr. Susan Love's Breast Book*. Reading: Addison-Wesley.

McGinn, K. A. 1987. *Keeping Abreast*. Palo Alto: Bull Publishing.

References Cited

Introduction

Sutherland, H. J., H. A. Llewellyn-Thomas, G. A. Lockwood, et al. 1989. "Cancer Patients: Their Desire for Information and Participation in Treatment Decisions." *Journal of the Royal Society of Medicine* 82:260–263.

Chapter 1

Kelly, P. T. 1980. "Counselling Needs of Women with a Maternal History of Breast Cancer." *Patient Counselling and Health Education* 2:118–124.

Lichtman, R. R., S. E. Taylor, J. V. Wood, et al. 1984. "Relations with Children After Breast Cancer: The Mother-Daughter Relationship at Risk." *Journal of Psychosocial Oncology* 2:1–19.

Chapter 2

Cook, R. R. 1989. "The Role of 'Negative' Epidemiology Data in the Evaluation of Risk." *Regulatory Toxicology and Pharmacology* 9: 44–52.

Feinstein, A. R. 1988. "Scientific Standards in Epidemiologic Studies of the Menace of Daily Life." *Science* 242:1257–1263.

Hill, A. B. 1971. *Principles of Medical Statistics*. New York: Oxford University Press.

Lilienfeld, A. M. 1976. *Foundations of Epidemiology*. New York: Oxford University Press.

Nomura, A. M., J. Lee, L. Kolonel, and T. Hirohata. 1984. "Breast Cancer in Two Populations with Different Levels of Risk for the Disease." *American Journal of Epidemiology* 119:496–502.

Seidman, Herbert. 1977. "Screening for Breast Cancer in Younger Women: Life Expectancy Gains and Losses." *Ca—A Cancer Journal for Clinicians* 27:66–87.

Chapter 3

Gump, F. E. 1987. "In Situ Cancers." In *Breast Disease*, edited by J. R. Harris, I. C. Henderson, S. Hellman, et al. Philadelphia: J. B. Lippincott.

Haagensen, C. D. 1986. *Diseases of the Breast*. Philadelphia: W. B. Saunders.

Lagios, M. D. 1990. "Duct Carcinoma In Situ." *Surgical Clinics of North America* 70:853–871.

Lagios, M. D., F. K. Margolin, P. R. Westdahl, and M. K. Rose. 1989. "Mammographically Detected Duct Carcinoma In Situ." *Cancer* 63:618–624.

Page, D. L., W. D. Dupont, L. W. Rogers, et al. 1985. "Atypical Hyperplastic Lesions of the Female Breast." *Cancer* 55:2698–2708.

———. 1982. "Intraductal Carcinoma of the Breast: Follow-up After Biopsy Only." *Cancer* 49:751–758.

Rosen, P. P., D. W. Braun, B. Lyngholm, et al. 1981. "Lobular Carcinoma In Situ of the Breast." *Cancer* 47:813–819.

Rosen, P. P., P. H. Lieberman, D. W. Braun, et al. 1978. "Lobular Carcinoma In Situ of the Breast." *American Journal of Surgical Pathology* 2:225–251.

Chapter 4

Adami, Hans-Olov, A. Rimsten, B. Stenkvist, et al. 1978. "Reproductive History and Risk of Breast Cancer." *Cancer* 41:747–757.

Adelstein, Arthur, and G. White. 1976. "Alcoholism and Mortality." *Population Trends* 6:7–13.

Anderson, D. E., and M. D. Badzioch. 1989. "Combined Effect of Family History and Reproductive Factors on Breast Cancer Risk." *Cancer* 63:349–353.

Brinton, L. A., R. Hoover, and J. F. Fraumeni. 1982. "Interaction of Familial and Hormonal Risk Factors for Breast Cancer." *Journal of the National Cancer Institute* 69:817–822.

Brinton, L. A., R. R. Williams, R. N. Hoover, et al. 1979. "Breast Cancer Risk Factors Among Screening Program Participants." *Journal of the National Cancer Institute* 62:37–44.

Brownson, R. C., C. W. Blackwell, D. K. Pearson, et al. 1988. "Risk of Breast Cancer in Relation to Cigarette Smoking." *Archives of Internal Medicine* 148:140–144.

Bulbrook, R. D. 1976. "Endocrine Status of Women with an Enhanced Risk of Breast Cancer." In *Breast Cancer: Trends in Research and Treatment*, edited by J. C. Heuson, W. H. Mattheiem, and M. Rozencweig. New York: Raven Press.

Cohen, L. A. 1986. "Dietary Fat and Mammary Cancer." In *Diet, Nutrition, and Cancer: A Critical Evaluation*, edited by B. S. Reddy and L. A. Cohen. Vol. 1. Boca Raton, Fla.: CRC Press.

Cowan, L. D., L. Gordis, J. A. Tonascia, et al. 1981. "Breast Cancer Incidence in Women with a History of Progesterone Deficiency." *American Journal of Epidemiology* 114:209–217.

Dattore, P. J., F. C. Shontz, and L. Coyne. 1980. "Premorbid Personality Differentiation of Cancer and Non-cancer Groups: A Test of the Hypothesis of Cancer Proneness." *Journal of Consulting and Clinical Psychology* 48:388–394.

Fox, B. H. 1983. "Current Theory of Psychogenic Effects on Cancer Incidence and Prognosis." *Journal of Psychosocial Oncology* 1:17–31.

Gail, M. H., L. A. Brinton, D. P. Byar, et al. 1989. "Projecting Individualized Probabilities of Developing Breast Cancer for White Females Who Are Being Examined Annually." *Journal of the National Cancer Institute* 81:1879–1886.

Graf, Ernst, and J. W. Eaton, 1985. "Dietary Suppression of Colonic Cancer." *Cancer* 56:717–718.

Graham, Saxon, J. Marshall, and C. Mettlen. 1982. "Diet in the Epidemiology of Breast Cancer." *American Journal of Epidemiology* 116:68–75.

Haagensen, C. D., C. Bodian, and D. E. Haagensen. 1981. *Breast Carcinoma Risk and Detection*. Philadelphia: W. B. Saunders.

Hahn, R. C. and D. B. Petitti. 1988. "Minnesota Multiphasic Personality Inventory-rated Depression and the Incidence of Breast Cancer." *Cancer* 61:845–848.

Harvey, E. B., C. Schairer, L. A. Brinton, et al. 1987. "Alcohol Consumption and Breast Cancer." *Journal of the National Cancer Institute* 78:657–661.

Henderson, B. E., D. Powell, I. Rosario, et al. 1974. "An Epidemiologic Study of Breast Cancer." *Journal of the National Cancer Institute* 53:609–614.

Hirayama, Takeshi. 1978. "Epidemiology of Breast Cancer with Special Reference to the Role of Diet." *Preventive Medicine* 7:173–195.

Ip, Clement. 1980. "Ability of Dietary Fat to Overcome the Resistance of Mature Female Rats to 7,12-Dimethylbenz[a]anthracene-induced Mammary Tumorigenesis." *Cancer Research* 40: 2785–2789.

Jones, D. Y., A. Schatzkin, S. B. Green, et al. 1987. "Dietary Fat and Breast Cancer in the National Health and Nutrition Examination Survey I Epidemiologic Follow-up Study." *Journal of the National Cancer Institute* 79:465–471.

Kinlen, L. J. 1982. "Meat and Fat Consumption and Cancer Mortality: A Study of Strict Religious Orders in Britain." *Lancet* 1: 946–949.

MacMahon, Brian, P. Cole, T. M. Lin, et al. 1970. "Age at First Birth and Breast Cancer Risk." *Bulletin of the World Health Organization* 43:209–221.

McTiernan, Ann, and D. Thomas. 1986. "Evidence for a Protective Effect of Lactation on Risk of Breast Cancer in Young Women." *American Journal of Epidemiology* 124:353–358.

Paganini-Hill, Annlia, and R. K. Ross. 1983. "Breast Cancer and Alcohol Consumption and Risk of Breast Cancer." *Lancet* 2:724–726.

Phillips, R. L., L. Garfinkel, J. W. Kuzoma, et al. 1980. "Mortality Among California Seventh-Day Adventists for Selected Cancer Sites." *Journal of the National Cancer Institute* 65:1097–1107.

Priestman, T. J., S. G. Priestman, and C. Bradshaw. 1985. "Stress and Breast Cancer." *British Journal of Cancer* 51:493–498.

Ron, Elaine, B. Lunefeld, J. Menczer, et al. 1987. "Cancer Incidence in a Cohort of Infertile Women." *American Journal of Epidemiology* 125:780–790.

Salber, E. J., D. Trichopoulos, and B. MacMahon. 1969. "Lactation and Reproductive Histories of Breast Cancer Patients in Boston, 1965–1966." *Journal of the National Cancer Institute* 43:1013–1024.

Sklar, L. S., and H. Anisman. 1981. "Stress and Cancer." *Psychological Bulletin* 89:369–405.

Sontag, Susan. 1979. *Illness as Metaphor*. New York: Vintage Books.

Stavraky, Kathleen, and S. Emmons, 1974. "Breast Cancer in Premenopausal and Postmenopausal Women." *Journal of the National Cancer Institute* 53:647–654.

Thomas, C. B., K. R. Duszynski, and J. W. Shaffer. 1979. "Family Attributes Reported in Youth as Potential Predictors of Cancer." *Psychosomatic Medicine* 41:287–302.

Trichopoulos, Dimitrios, B. MacMahon, and P. Cole. 1972. "Menopause and Breast Cancer Risk." *Journal of the National Cancer Society* 48:605–613.

Webster, L. A., P. M. Layde, P. A. Wingo, et al. 1983. "Alcohol Consumption and Risk of Breast Cancer." *Lancet* 2:724–726.

Willett, W. C., M. J. Stampfer, G. A. Colditz, et al. 1987a. "Dietary Fat and the Risk of Breast Cancer." *New England Journal of Medicine* 316:22–28.

———. 1987b. "Moderate Alcohol Consumption and the Risk of Breast Cancer." *New England Journal of Medicine* 316:1174–1180.

Wynder, E. L., F. A. MacCormack, and S. D. Stillman. 1978. "The Epidemiology of Breast Cancer in 785 United States Caucasian Women." *Cancer* 41:2341–2354.

Wynder, E. L., D. P. Rose, and L. A. Cohen. 1986. "Diet and Breast Cancer in Causation and Therapy." *Cancer* 58(Suppl.):1804–1813.

Yuasa, Shu, and Brian MacMahon. 1970. "Lactation and Reproductive Histories of Breast Cancer Patients in Tokyo, Japan." *Bulletin of the World Health Organization* 42:195–204.

Chapter 5

Adess, Nancy, K. Brown, and S. Hackett. 1983. *Fertility and Pregnancy Guide for DES Daughters and Sons*. New York: DES Action National.

Astedt, Birger. 1987. "Cancer and Other Risk Factors with Estrogen Replacement." *Acta Obstet Gynecologica Scandinavica Suppl* 140: 46–51.

Bayliss, Richard, Cyril Clarke, and A. G. Whitfield. 1987. "Problems in Comparative Longevity." *Journal of the Royal College of Physicians, London* 21:134–139.

Beral, Valerie, and L. Colwell. 1980. "Randomised Trial of High Doses of Stilboestrol and Ethisterone in Pregnancy: Long-term Follow-up of Mothers." *British Medical Journal* 281:1098–1101.

Bergkvist, Leif, H.-O. Adami, I. Persson, et al. 1989. "The Risk of

Breast Cancer After Estrogen and Estrogen-progestin Replacement." *New England Journal of Medicine* 321:293–297.

Bibbo, Marluce, W. M. Haenszel, and G. L. Wied. 1978. "A Twenty-five Year Follow-up Study of Women Exposed to Diethylstilbestrol During Pregnancy." *New England Journal of Medicine* 298: 763–767.

Brian, D. D., B. C. Tilley, and D. R. Labarthe. 1980. "Breast Cancer in DES-exposed Mothers." *Mayo Clinic Proceedings* 55:89–93.

Brinton, L. A., R. Hoover, and J. F. Fraumeni. 1986. "Menopausal Oestrogens and Breast Cancer Risk: An Expanded Case-control Study." *British Journal of Cancer* 54:825–832.

Bush, T. L., L. D. Cowan, E. Barrett-Connor, et al. 1983. "Estrogen Use and All-cause Mortality: Preliminary Results from the Lipid Research Clinics Program Follow-up Study." *Journal of American Medical Association* 249:903–906.

Chilvers, Clair, K. McPherson, J. Peto, et al. 1989. "Oral Contraceptive Use and Breast Cancer Risk in Young Women." *Lancet* (May 6): 973–982.

Feinstein, A. R. 1988. "Scientific Standards in Epidemiologic Studies of the Menace of Daily Life." *Science* 242:1257–1263.

Gordon, Tavia. 1978. "Menopause and Coronary Heart Disease: The Framingham Study." *Annals of Internal Medicine* 89:157–161.

Greenberg, E. R., A. B. Barnes, L. Resseguie, et al. 1984. "Breast Cancer in Mothers Given Diethylstilbestrol in Pregnancy." *New England Journal of Medicine* 311:1393–1398.

Hadjimichael, D. C., J. W. Meigs, and F. W. Falcier. 1984. "Cancer Risk Among Women Exposed to Exogenous Estrogens During Pregnancy." *Journal of the National Cancer Institute* 73:831–834.

Henderson, B. E., A. Paganini-Hill, and R. K. Ross. 1988. "Estrogen Replacement Therapy and Protection from Acute Myocardial Infarction." *American Journal of Obstetrics and Gynecology* 159: 312–317.

Herbst, A. L., S. Anderson, M. Hubby, et al. 1986. "Risk Factors for the Development of Diethylstilbestrol-associated Clear Cell Adenocarcinoma: A Case-control Study." *American Journal of Obstetrics and Gynecology* 154:14–22.

Hoover, Robert, L. A. Gray, P. Cole, et al. 1976. "Menopausal Estrogens and Breast Cancer." *New England Journal of Medicine* 295: 401–405.

Hunt, Kathryn, Martin Vessey, Klim McPherson, et al. 1987. "Long-term Surveillance of Mortality and Cancer Incidence in Women Receiving Hormone Replacement Therapy." *British Journal of Obstetrics and Gynecology* 94:620–635.

Hutchinson, T. A., S. M. Polansky, and A. D. Feinstein. 1979. "Postmenopausal Estrogens Protect Against Fractures of Hip and Distal Radius." *Lancet* 2:705–709.

Kaufman, D. W., D. R. Miller, L. Rosenberg, et al. 1984. "Noncontraceptive Estrogen Use and the Risk of Breast Cancer." *Journal of American Medical Association* 252:63–67.

Kay, C. R., and P. C. Hannaford. 1988. "Breast Cancer and the Pill—A Further Report from the Royal College of General Practioners' Oral Contraceptive Study." *British Journal of Cancer* 58:675–680.

Konicki, A. M. 1985. "Physical and Psychological Effects of DES on Exposed Offspring." *Cancer Nursing* 8:233–237.

Krieger, Nancy, J. L. Kelsey, T. R. Holford, et al. 1982. "An Epidemiological Study of Hip Fracture in Post-menopausal Women." *American Journal of Epidemiology* 116:141–148.

Paganini-Hill, Annlia, R. K. Ross, and B. E. Henderson. 1988. "Postmenopausal Oestrogen Treatment and Stroke: A Prospective Study." *British Medical Journal* 297:519–522.

Paul, Charlotte, D.C.G. Skegy, G.F.S. Spears, et al. 1986. "Oral Contraceptives and Breast Cancer: A National Study." *British Medical Journal* 293:723–726.

Rosner, Dutzu, and W. W. Lane. 1986. "Oral Contraceptive Use Has No Adverse Effect on the Prognosis of Breast Cancer." *Cancer* 57:591–596.

Sattin, R. W., G. L. Rubin, P. A. Wingo, et al. 1986. "Oral-contraceptive Use and the Risk of Breast Cancer." *New England Journal of Medicine* 315:405–411.

Shapiro, Samuel. 1986. "Oral Contraceptives—Time to Take Stock." *New England Journal of Medicine* 315:450–451.

Silverberg, Edwin, and J. A. Lubera. 1983. "Cancer Statistics, 1983." *Ca—A Cancer Journal for Clinicians* 33:2–8.

Stadel, B. V., G. L. Rubin, L. A. Webster, et al. 1985. "Oral Contraceptives and Breast Cancer in Young Women." *Lancet* (Nov. 2):970–973.

Stampfer, M. J., W. C. Willett, G. A. Colditz, et al. 1985. "A Prospective Study of Postmenopausal Estrogen Therapy and Coronary Heart Disease. *New England Journal of Medicine* 313:1044–1049.

Weiss, N. J., C. L. Ure, J. H. Ballard, et al. 1980. "Decreased Risk of

Fractures of the Hip and Lower Forearm with Post-menopausal Use of Estrogen." *New England Journal of Medicine* 303:1195–1198.

Wilson, P.W.F., R. J. Garrison, and W. P. Castelli. 1985. "Post-menopausal Estrogen Use, Cigarette Smoking, and Cardiovascular Morbidity in Women Over 50: The Framingham Study." *New England Journal of Medicine* 313:1038–1043.

Wingo, P. A., P. M. Layde, N. C. Lee, et al. 1987. "The Risk of Breast Cancer in Postmenopausal Women Who Have Used Estrogen Replacement Therapy." *Journal of the American Medical Association* 257:209–215.

Chapter 6

Anderson, D. E., and M. D. Badzioch. 1985. "Risk of Familial Breast Cancer." *Cancer* 56:383–387.

Claus, E. B., N. J. Risch, and W. D. Thompson. 1990. "Age at Onset as an Indicator of Familial Risk of Breast Cancer." *American Journal of Epidemiology* 131:961–972.

Henderson, B. E., V. R. Gerkins, M. C. Pike, et al. 1977. "Endocrine Function and Breast Cancer," in J. J. Mulvihill, R. W. Miller, and J. F. Fraumeni, Jr., eds., *The Genetics of Human Cancer*. New York: Raven Press.

Knudson, A. G. 1986. "Genetics of Human Cancer." *Annual Review of Genetics* 20:231–251.

———. 1971. "Mutation and Cancer: Statistical Study of Retinoblastoma." *Proceedings of the National Academy of Science* 68:820–823.

Lynch, H. T. 1981. *Genetics and Breast Cancer*. New York: Van Nostrand Reinhold.

Macklin, M. T. 1959. "Comparison of the Number of Breast Cancer Deaths Observed in Relatives of Breast Cancer Patients, and the Number Expected on the Basis of Mortality Rates." *Journal of the National Cancer Institute* 22:927–951.

Murphree, A. L., and W. F. Benedict. 1984. "Retinoblastoma: Clues to Human Oncogenesis," *Science* 223:1028–1033.

Ottman, Ruth, M. C. Pike, M.-C. King, et al. 1983. "Practical Guide for Estimating Risk for Familial Breast Cancer." *Lancet* (Sept. 3):556–558.

Schwartz, A. G., M.-C. King, S. H. Belle, et al. 1985. "Risk of Breast

Cancer to Relatives of Young Breast Cancer Patients." *Journal of the National Cancer Institute* 75:665–668.
Taylor, J. A. 1989. "Oncogenes and Their Applications in Epidemiologic Studies." *American Journal of Epidemiology* 130:6–13.

Chapter 7

Donegan, W. L. and J. S. Spratt. 1979. *Cancer of the Breast.* Philadelphia: W. B. Saunders.
Fisher, Bernard, N. H. Slack, and I. D. Bross. 1969. "Cancer of the Breast: Size of Neoplasm and Prognosis." *Cancer* 24:1071–1080.
Fletcher, S. W., M. S. O'Malley, and L. A. Bunce. 1985. "Physicians' Abilities to Detect Lumps in Silicone Breast Models." *Journal of the American Medical Association* 253:2224–2228.
Habbema, J.D.F., G. J. van Oostmarssen, D. van Putten, et al. 1986. "Age-specific Reduction in Breast Cancer Mortality by Screening: An Analysis of the Results of the Health Insurance Plan of Greater New York Study." *Journal of the National Cancer Institute* 77:317–320.
Letton, A. H., and E. M. Mason. 1986. "Routine Breast Screening." *Annals of Surgery* 203:470–473.
Margolin, F. R., and M. D. Lagios. 1986. "Mammographic Detection of Early Breast Cancer." *Western Journal of Medicine* 144:46–48.
Nemoto, T., N. Natarajan, C. R. Smart, et al. 1982. "Patterns of Breast Cancer Detection in the United States." *Journal of Surgical Oncology* 21:183–188.
Shapiro, Samuel. 1989. "Determining the Efficacy of Breast Cancer Screening." *Cancer* 63:1873–1880.
Tabar, L., C.J.G. Fagerberg, A. Gad, et al. 1985. "Reduction in Mortality from Breast Cancer After Mass Screening with Mammography." *Lancet* (April 13):829–832.
Yang, J. H., N. H. Slack, and T. Nemoto. 1987. "Effect of Axillary Nodal Status on the Long-term Survival Following Mastectomy for Breast Carcinoma: Nodal Metastases May Not Always Suggest Systemic Disease." *Journal of Surgical Oncology* 36:243–248.

Index